Heal yourself with

Flowers

and other essences

"When you no longer know how to go further,
let the plants tell you — learn the language of the flowers."

Albert Steffen

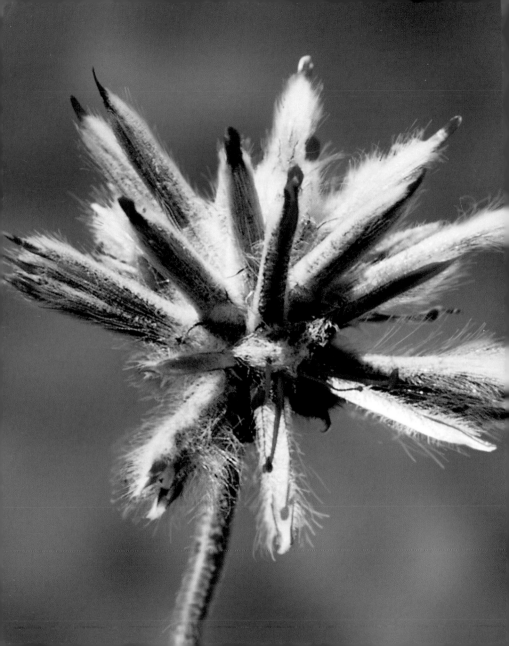

Heal yourself with
Flowers
and other essences

NIKKI BRADFORD

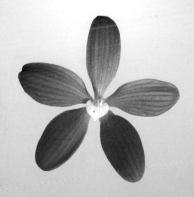

QUADRILLE

EDITORIAL CONSULTANTS, BETH TYERS AND ROSE TITCHINER

This book is a reference work, and is not intended to diagnose, prescribe, prevent, or treat disease. The information it offers is not considered to be a replacement for consultation with an appropriate licensed medical healthcare professional.

This edition first published in 2007 by Quadrille Publishing Ltd
Alhambra House, 27–31 Charing Cross Road,
London WC2H 0LS

Project editor Anne Furniss
Design Ros Holder
Picture research Samantha Rolfe
Illustration Richard Rockwood
Production Rebecca Short, Vincent Smith

British Library Cataloguing in Publication Data
A catalogue record for this book is available from the British Library

ISBN: 978 184400 428 7
Printed and bound in Singapore

10 9 8 7 6 5 4 3 2 1

Contents

Introducing essences

Essence therapy is the most exciting and important new form of complementary medicine to emerge in the last 100 years. It is also perfect for the 21st century's unique challenges, upheavals, and uncertainties, for it combines power with subtlety, and simple hands-on, can-do practicality with the catalyst for personal development.

Simple enough for anyone to use and gentle enough to be given to babies, essences can be so effective that they are increasingly being used in hospital pain clinics, children's homes, and hospices. Child psychotherapists, psychologists, progressive gynecologists, and even vets are beginning to offer these remedies, as many complementary therapists including osteopaths, homeopaths, acupuncturists, and healers have done for some time. Essences are also increasingly being bought and used to great effect by the general public for themselves, their families, and their friends.

Where do essences come from?
The first modern ones were developed by a British physician called Dr. Edward Bach more than 70 years ago, perhaps the best known being Rescue Remedy. However, there is now an explosion of remarkable new essence ranges emerging worldwide — from the Australian outback to the slopes of the Himalayas; from the foothills of America's Sierra Nevada, to the southern tip of Africa. This rapidly developing form of therapy is an international phenomenon.

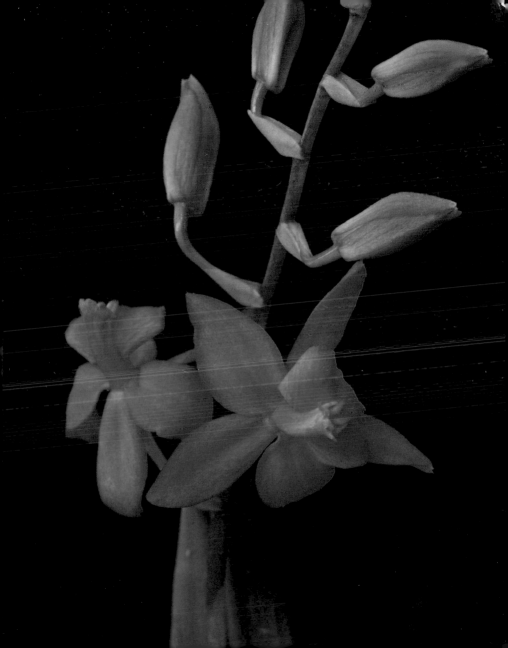

What is in them?

Essences are a type of vibrational medicine (see page 12) in the form of very diluted healing tinctures containing the energy imprint of certain beneficial natural substances. Most are made from plants, but there are many other sources, including gems and animal energy (see pages 293–301). They are very different from aromatherapy's essential oils, for those are the concentrated distillations of plants, while these are drawn from the energy of the plant or other substance. And while there are similarities with homeopathy, essences are made differently and work as much on the spiritual part of the mind-body-spirit system that makes up every human being, as on the emotions and the physical body.

What do they do?

Essence therapy can be used on an immediate, practical level for physical problems as diverse as tiredness, backache, low energy, ill temper, premenstrual syndrome (PMS), lack of sex drive, and poor sleep. But it can also be a subtle and gentle tool for someone who appears well and seems to have their life running as they would wish, yet has a sense that somehow, somewhere, there is an important element missing that they cannot quite put their finger on.

Essences never push. What they will do is work gently yet powerfully, pointing the way forward and helping to bring about change for the better — if you are ready for it, and if it is what you truly want.

A single essence may have several different properties, and you absorb the one(s) you need. Certain essences that are made from the same plant but by different people in different parts of the world may also have different qualities, because much depends on the maker, the place where the plant is grown and the characteristics perceived by the maker while they produce the essence.

These remedies can work fast. Sometimes their effect is immediate, often a change occurs within a few days, and the longest it will take for you to notice the difference is a couple of weeks. They are entirely safe and there are no recorded side effects.

How do you take them?

Essences are taken as droplets placed under your tongue or in water, usually three to four times daily. They are often taken singly, but several essences can be mixed together in combinations. These mixtures generally contain between three and eight essences, each addressing a particular aspect of the same issue. If you are not sure which single essence to choose, a good ready-made combination can be an excellent place to start.

Essences are also effective when added to baths and massage creams, misted via sprays around a room, or applied directly to the skin.

How do they work?

It is easier to understand how and why essences work if you look at an energy map that shows what is inside and around your physical body.

The diagram on the following page shows your seven main energy centers, or chakras, plus the subtle (fine) energy layers surrounding you. If there is a blockage, trauma, or weakness (often caused by prolonged psychological distress) in any one or more of these chakras, it may

AREA OF CONNECTION	CHAKRA	PROBLEM AREAS
Spiritual awareness, connection with God/Buddha/Source.	CROWN	Lack of meaning in life, lost, alienated.
Intuition, clarity of thought.	THIRD EYE	Eye disorders, headaches.
Communication, speaking/listening/ opinions.	THROAT	Laryngitis, thyroid and throat diseases.
Love of all types, the emotions, storing hurt and sadness.	HEART	Heart, lung, and breast disorders.
Personal identity/ power, self-esteem, energy.	SOLAR PLEXUS	Ulcers, low confidence, weak immune system.
Sexuality, sensuality, reproduction, creativity.	SACRAL	Pelvic and reproductive disorders, lack of libido.
Feeling safe, belonging.	BASE	Feeling threatened, spaced out, anxious.

Chakra chart

eventually produce a physical problem in the area of the body which that chakra usually supplies with energy.

This doesn't mean that genetics, infections, poor nutrition, or environmental toxins are not important factors in illness, because they are. What it does mean is that a low or restricted energy flow through a chakra can create a "weak link" in its corresponding physical body part, which then determines where illness shows up. For example, a blockage in the throat chakra caused by bottling up what you need to say may eventually produce chronic, hard-to-treat laryngitis which might have no obvious medical cause.

There are thought to be seven subtle-energy bodies curled around you like the layers of an onion, the first of which shows up clearly on Kirlian photography as a layer of light. These energy layers merge together to form the aura. Your aura is, in fact, a continuation of your physical body — effectively, your body and aura are one, but simply made from different types of energy.

Essences are thought to be able to help with physical problems, too, on the basis that if something can affect the mind or spirit, it can affect the body via these routes as well — hence mind-body-spirit, or holistic, medicine. Essences are true mind-body-spirit remedies, as they operate by first entering the aura, where they work on an emotional (mind) and spiritual level. Then, because there is no separation between those aspects of you and your solid body, they can go on to affect you physically, and may do so very swiftly.

Vibrational medicine

"They [essences] cure, not by attacking the disease, but by flooding our bodies with the vibrations of our higher nature, in the presence of which disease melts away as snow in the sunshine."   Dr. Edward Bach

Vibrational medicine uses positive energy instead of solid matter to restore wellbeing. Homeopathy, radionics, color, light, and sound therapies, spiritual healing and essence therapy are all forms of vibrational medicine. A vibrational remedy's active ingredient is a positive energy imprint instead of a pharmaceutical drug, or other conventional medicinal substance such as a herb or vitamin.

An essence is the energy imprint of something therapeutic, held and preserved in pure water. In this context, energy could be described as something's life force, the special "feel" of it, or, if it is a place, its atmosphere. Essences can be made from the energy of many different things including plants, gems, weather conditions, places, and animals (though no animal is ever harmed, or even touched): see page 17.

The hidden messages of water

Ongoing scientific research supports the idea that water takes on and maintains energy imprints. Homeopathy, in which remedies are also made by capturing energy imprints in water, is backed by hundreds of published clinical trials confirming it works. Further, investigations supporting the concept of imprinting energy into water have been carried out by scientists in Japan, and also by Dr. Lee H. Lorenzen at the

University of California, Berkeley. They all took water samples from different sources — pure springs, polluted lakes, even inner-city tap water — froze it, and then examined the resulting snowflake patterns. Those from pure sources were uniform and beautiful, those from polluted origins, deformed. Further experiments showed that the energy of music and even written phrases also radically altered the snowflake shapes. Paper bearing the words "Thank You" in several languages was placed on the water samples and produced symmetrical patterns, while "You Make Me Sick" created malformed, unfinished ones.

The scientific explanation

The theory for vibrational medicine is based on quantum physics, the study of subatomic particles. Many consider this to be the point where science meets spirituality, and explains why this type of medicine works.

Quantum law states that all matter vibrates, that each type does so at its own special frequency or rate, and that it is this vibrational frequency that determines the physical form the matter takes — suggesting that the only difference between a brick and a flower essence is the frequency at which it is vibrating. This is what Albert Einstein meant when he said that energy and matter are just two different forms of the same thing.

Following on from this idea, that existence is essentially a matter of vibrational frequency, it is now thought that vibrational medicine works because illness often results when our proper vibrational rates are disrupted. These disruptions can be corrected by exposing them to the correct, or healthy, rates that will stimulate healing. Essence therapy is one effective way of restoring a healthy vibrational rate to the human system.

Essences in medicine

Essences may be gentle, but they can also be so powerful that hospitals and clinics worldwide are starting to use them for problems ranging from severe burns and chronic pain to drug addiction and cancer (see below). And today's new generation of remedies are gaining respect from the medical establishment in a way that the original Bach Flower Remedies, developed 70 years ago, and still much loved, never really have.

This may be because many of the new essences appear deeper-acting and longer-lasting. No one has a definitive answer as to why this might be, but one theory is that nature shows humans what they need at exactly the right time, producing these things only when we are ready for them. If this is so, the increased power of the new essences is completely appropriate, for we are now facing global problems and personal challenges that did not exist in Dr. Bach's time — challenges that his remedies were never designed to deal with.

* **Swiss medical charity Green Cross** uses Australian Bush Flower Essences' Electro Essence with spirulina extract in Belarus to treat child victims of Chernobyl, working with the worst cases whose radiation levels were extreme. Levels have dropped by between one-third and one-half so far, and still counting. The same range has a major ongoing double-blind placebo trial in Australia with its She Oak for hormonal rebalancing.

* **In São Paulo, Brazil**, Dr. Katia Kuchler has carried out a trial with the local health departments using Peach Flowered Tea-Tree to treat insulin-dependent diabetes, noting a significant reduction in glucose levels, pain, infection, and insomnia. The University Hospital in São Paulo uses Fireweed in its burns unit. Several institutional homes for street children use Ararêtama essences for health and emotional problems, especially low self-esteem. In the same city, Hospital São Camilo and the University Hospital now use remedies by Living Essences of Australia (LEA).

* **In the United States**, the Texas Cancer Care Center in Fort Worth and the Baylor Medical Center in Dallas have cancer-support programs that use the Petite Fleur range, particularly for vomiting, nausea, anxiety, and stress.

* **In Western Australia**, hospitals such as the Royal Perth, pain clinics, rehabilitation centers, nursing homes, and the South Eastern Drug & Alcohol Rehabilitation Service in Victoria use LEA remedies. In 2001, research with heroin addicts found that 80% relapsed quickly after treatment, but this dropped to 7% for those taking an essence mixture.

* **Italian research** by pediatrician Dr. S. Calzolari, released in 1999 after studying 417 children for three years, concluded that Bach flower remedies were very effective in helping them deal with emotional difficulties. Another trial, conducted by Drs. D'Auria and Pezza, suggested that Bach remedies help control psychological aspects of pain.

* **Japan** uses its own and other international ranges at centers such as the Niwa Clinic in Tokyo and the Ando Clinic in Chiba-ken.

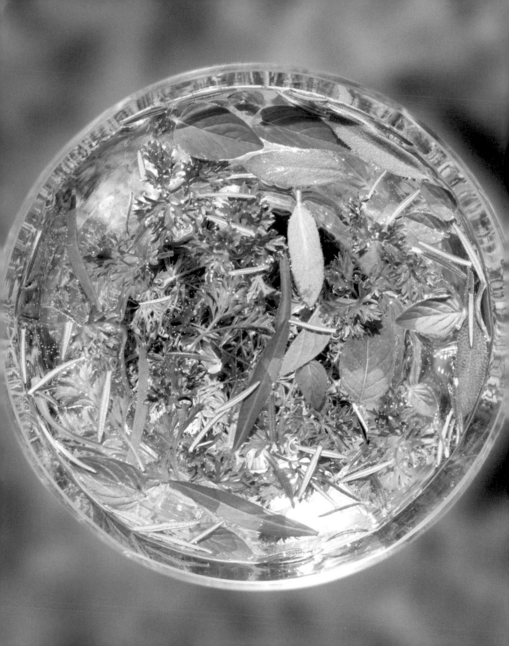

How an essence is made

When an essence is made, the nature or "personality" and power of the plant, gem, animal, or environment concerned (its unique signature energy and vibrational rate) are transferred into water. A healing substance, such as organically grown flowers, is placed in a bowl of pure water and left in the sunlight for several hours before being gently removed. What remains behind is the "mother tincture," a mixture of captured therapeutic energy and water. The result is a bit like a homeopathic remedy — a substance turbocharged with the energy of that living thing or place, which, while having no trace of its ingredients detectable by ordinary measuring devices, will nevertheless have the ability to affect in a profound and positive way whoever takes it.

Several drops of this mother tincture are then added to any size bottle up to 30ml containing 2/3 brandy (or glycerine or saline solution) and 1/3 pure water, resulting in the "stock" bottles available to buy from health and esoteric shops or by mail order.

Essences take on the feel of their place of origin (and their developer's personality) as well. For example, the Bush range from the Australian outback, where the flora contains ancient, grounded Aboriginal energy, has many essences for physical problems. The steamy Brazilian rainforests produce many remedies addressing fertility, sexuality, and exuberance. The flowers of the high Himalayas provide a collection that is meditational and spiritual, while the Alaskan wilderness essences' power and purity echo their pristine environment, and are excellent for personal development and space clearing.

How to choose essences

There are thousands of essences available from over 200 ranges made all over the world. With such a choice, how can you know which to pick? Luckily, it's pretty straightforward — a therapy does not need to be complicated in order to be effective. While wonderfully easy to use, essences are also "intelligent," self-adjusting healing tinctures which seem to steer you toward choosing those you need. You can't get it wrong — if the essence is not what's needed, it will simply have no effect.

When choosing your remedy, go with what feels right. As parenting guru Dr. Benjamin Spock used to tell mothers and fathers: "Trust yourself. You know more than you think." Below are some self-help methods that may be useful. Many people use one method to make an initial choice, then another to double-check it.

Use the Index of Symptoms

The quickest and easiest approach is to look up the problem or issue that concerns you in the Index of Symptoms on page 282. This will point you to the best relevant essences in this book, chosen from 18 ranges. Then turn to the entries for the suggested essences, reading the "– (negative) indications" (difficulties the essence can help with), the "+ effects" (benefits/results of using the essence), and the full comments. Based on this information, and on your own intuition, decide which essence is for you.

Look at essence photographs

Essences send out promptings ("Choose me!") that people can register subliminally, as can pictures of the plants from which they were made (take a look at those in this book). If you are investigating one particular range in depth, some essence makers offer books with photographs of the plants, places, or animals from whose energies their particular essences were made; others produce packs of picture cards to help you.

Finger testing

This is a simplified form of the muscle-testing technique used by kinesiologists. Link the tip of your little finger and the tip of your thumb on your non-dominant hand, then:

* If you already have a hunch about what the answer may be, empty your mind or it may influence the result.

* Ask your question, keeping it simple and clear: for example, "Will Mountain Lion essence improve my confidence?"

* Try to break the thumb/finger circuit by pulling them apart with your other hand. It will hold firm for a "Yes," and break easily for a "No."

Dowsing and other techniques

Dowsing is an ancient divining technique that picks up on the vibrational frequencies or messages sent out by all forms of matter. It involves using a pendulum to get a yes/no answer. With practice, many people can dowse accurately to choose the essences they need.

How to take essences

When you have chosen your essence, follow the manufacturer's recommended dosage.

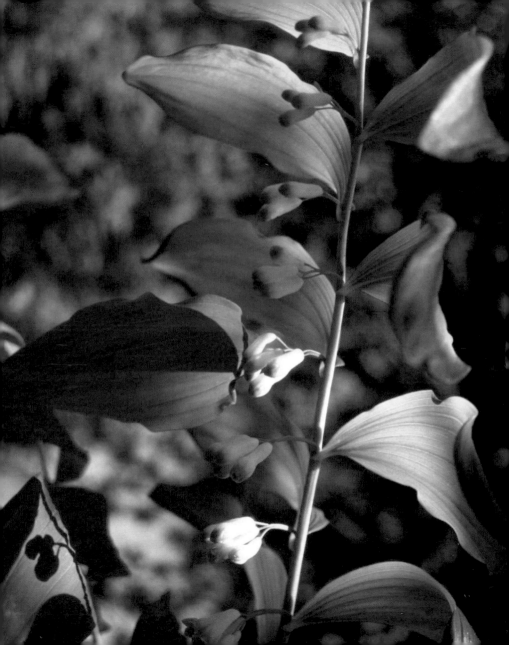

Relaxation

A certain amount of stress can be stimulating,
healthy, even fun — some would say it's
positively necessary to keep life interesting. As
the normal human response to challenge, stress
creates a buzz that acts as a positive catalyst for
swift, decisive action or creative ideas. However,
excessively high stress levels are now endemic
worldwide, and since research by Harvard
Medical School has suggested that up to 90%
of modern disorders may be stress-related,
finding ways to both reduce it and mediate our
own responses to it are excellent ways to help
safeguard health on all levels. If you can't see an
individual essence that addresses the way you
feel but would like something to help you calm
down, consider a good general combination
such as Relaxation and Harmony, or Tranquility.

SOLOMON'S SEAL

Solomon's Seal *(UK)*

— INDICATIONS

lots to do, but can never seem to finish things
bogged down by trivia
cannot settle to essential tasks
people see you as a soft touch and are using you
difficulty meditating, as your mind won't be still

+ EFFECTS

quietens your mind, helps you identify your own needs
prevents you from becoming so carried away by others' requests
reasserts control over your mind, making meditation easier
enables you to settle to the jobs you need to do
shows you that by doing less, you become more efficient

This is a great essence for the busy, busy mind — scourge of those who cannot meditate because thoughts are constantly chattering in their head. As the developer of this essence puts it: "Our minds should be our servants, not our masters. Solomon's Seal helps you reassert your rightful control, but it is rather like training an unruly dog — very worthwhile, but it may take an appreciable time." However, if you are stressed more because you feel as if you are on a treadmill and are permanently tired/wound up, try the soothing Fuji Cherry as well, or even instead.

Thini-A (BRA)

— INDICATIONS

insecurity about everything, producing excessive, repetitive thoughts

fear, anxiety, tension

anger

hypersensitivity

difficulty relaxing and opening up

+ EFFECTS

releases anxiety

relaxes the nervous system

dissipates tension

helps you feel lighter

enables you to live in the present

prevents you from obsessing over the future

This essence is made from the plant known as Spanish moss. It grows in the Brazilian rainforests, where it hangs in profusion from the branches of trees, forming long, draping garlands of grayish-green stems and leaves as fine as hair. Thini-A essence is especially good for using with bodywork therapies like massage to help a tense person relax — it can be added to massage creams or oils — and for encouraging both emotional and physical relaxation in women during childbirth.

Comfrey (S AF)

— INDICATIONS

nervous breakdown
nervous depletion/exhaustion
stress-related habits such as nail-biting, hair-tugging
emotional tension
irritability
panic or anxiety attacks

+ EFFECTS

calms you down
has a balancing effect
restores vitality
releases tension
encourages tranquility and serenity

Comfrey can be calming and supportive if you feel as though you've been driven right to the edge by stress, or are recovering from any type or degree of nervous breakdown. However, for committed, driven people — those whose response to stress is simply to do even more as they strive to be perfect — Dandelion as well or instead may be a better choice.

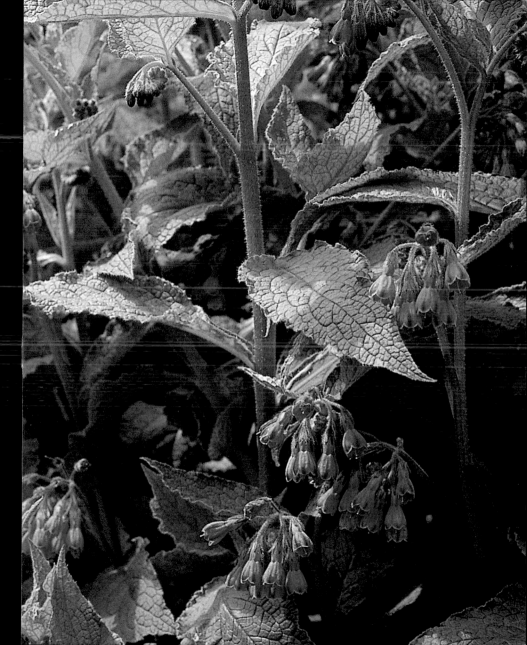

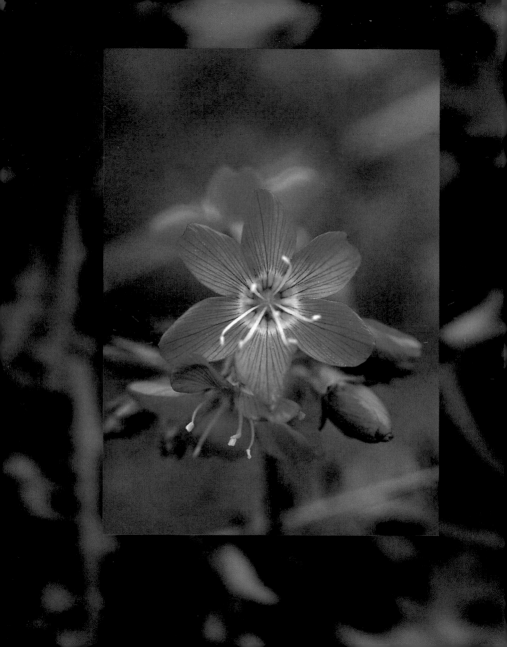

Jacob's Ladder (ALASKA)

− INDICATIONS

obsessive, self-imposed hypervigilance

controlling, manipulating

anxiety

insomnia

constant worrying over detail

tension in muscles

+ EFFECTS

enables you to let go of your obsessive need for control

helps you feel trust

promotes acceptance

encourages mental relaxation

This is the essence for those who feel that if they don't maintain their obsessive mental watchfulness, everything will fall apart. However, if you are caught in a powerful pattern of control and like to feel that you run the show, but also suffer from an eating disorder or digestive problems and struggle with a fragile sense of self-worth (perhaps stemming from childhood) consider Sea Palm (see page 35). This essence is also indicated if you can only release your tension when some external crisis brings you to a sudden halt: the scenario in which you only stop to take stock when metaphorically hit by a truck.

Plurk (Eire)

— INDICATIONS

desperate to succeed
stressed about things you have to do
under pressure to perform
snowed under
bored with work, and/or overwhelmed by the volume of it

+ EFFECTS

encourages you to stop taking things so seriously
helps you realize anew that life is also meant to be fun
enables you to ignore those who tell you otherwise
renews your sense of proportion about work

Great for children inundated with homework, or whose school or parents are trying to push them too hard, Plurk says what it means: Play and Work balance. It is helpful, too, for adults whose workplaces demand excessive commitment and that you give the company your all, 24/7. This essence also offers balance and support to women who are having to try extra-hard in male-dominated arenas like banking and certain areas of industry, where chauvinism and glass-ceiling thinking are still endemic.

Dragonfly (USA)

— INDICATIONS

need to relax — but just can't

difficulty sleeping

physically and mentally tense

anxious, worried

no time to slow down

+ EFFECTS

promotes rest

enables you to take time to relax

encourages letting go

makes it easier to lighten up

Dragonfly supports you in calming down, letting go, and resting comfortably after busy periods. It can be very helpful if you are self-employed, or cannot wind down at the end of the workday. For nurturing feelings of peace, calm, and stillness, also consider Dove — especially if you find you are often in conflict with others. Dove offers support to people who are under great stress, and is a good choice for whole families to take together during difficult times.

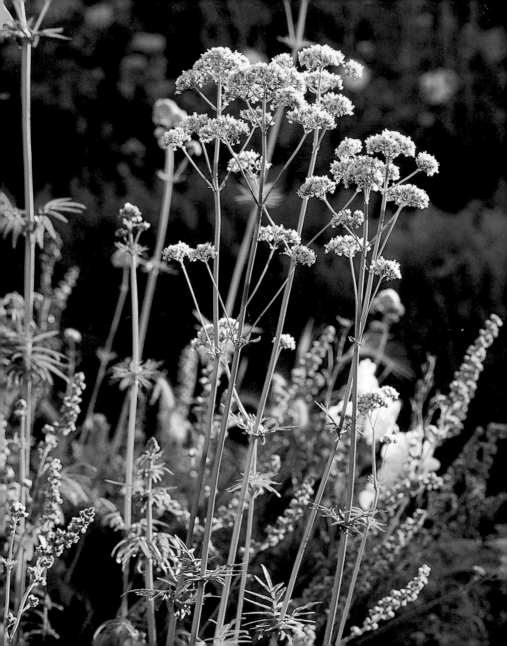

Valerian (UK)

— INDICATIONS

beguiled by the idea of being super-busy
for workaholics of all types
over-striving, stressed, and tense
for hurry and worry
lost sense of fun/humor
weighed down by responsibilities, whether self-induced or inescapable

+ EFFECTS

encourages contentment
stimulates spontaneity
increases pleasure and happiness in just "being"
creates a joyful appreciation of what you already have
enables you to laugh at yourself

This is an essence for anyone who overworks and finds it difficult to stop, or who has been captivated by the image of themselves as a hardworking, highly effective multitasker and is now stuck with it. If you can't help feeling that because there is always something that needs doing, there is no time for fun and play, Valerian is for you. It is also helpful where an overactive mind causes sleep problems: Perhaps you cannot get to sleep in the first place, or you wake in the small hours and that's it, for your mind simply starts up once again.

Black Eyed Susan (AUS)

— INDICATIONS

constantly expending energy and permanently on the go

often impatient

always striving

feeling stressed

finding it difficult to ask others to take on tasks for you

may suffer digestive problems

+ EFFECTS

promotes peace and calm

helps you slow down

invites you to turn inward and be still

encourages you to delegate more

helps you have more gentleness and sympathy for others

This is a great anti-hurry essence for fast-moving, quick-thinking people who try to do too much, and who often have several projects on the go simultaneously. Black Eyed Susan is a very urban remedy which helps speedy, 24/7 types slow down and find that still, balanced place within themselves that will help them cope better with fast-paced city living. However, if you are a major worrier, consider Crowea instead or as well, for it can help calm and center you, especially if, for example, you are getting nervous before a performance or business presentation.

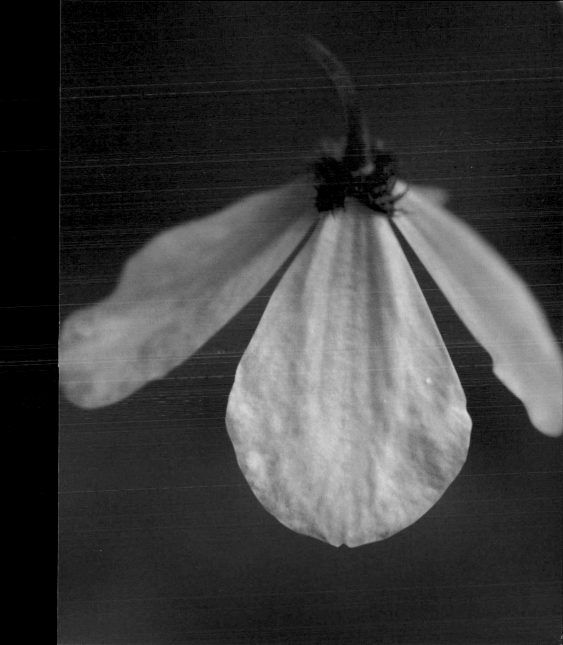

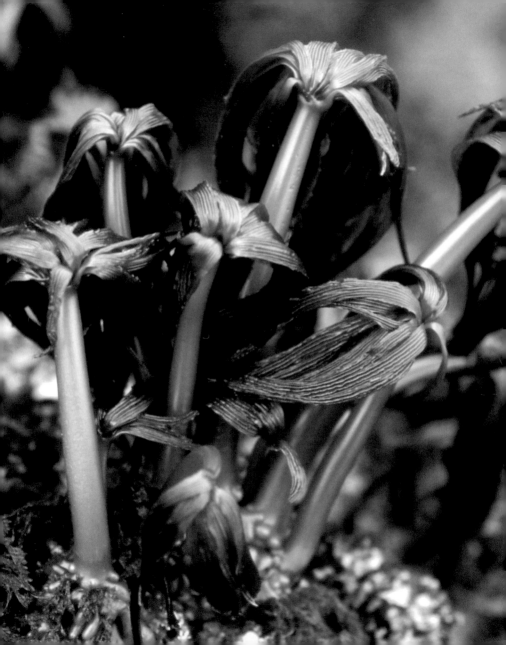

Sea Palm (CAN)

— INDICATIONS

rushing about, always doing things
caught in a hefty pattern of control
like to feel you are running the show
may not have enough time for relationships
low self-worth
may suffer digestive problems, or eating disorders

+ EFFECTS

balances a hurry-for-nothing attitude
allows life to flow more
encourages "allowing" — and just "be-ing"

This is the essence for those who never take the time to smell the flowers because they are always too busy pushing the river. Their very busyness can be a hindrance to success and also to meaningful relationships, while their need for control and constant activity can cause tension on both the physical and emotional levels. This is usually only released when that person is brought to a sudden halt by an external crisis — perhaps a breakdown in health or an "accident." Sea Palm people often crave nurturing and nourishment, both emotionally and physically, for they may have low self-worth stemming from feeling unloved, unwanted, or not good enough when they were children.

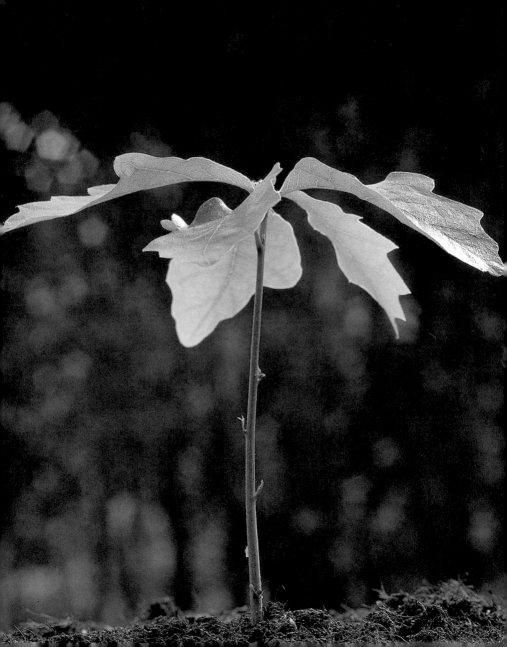

Energy

Tiredness is the most common health problem
there is. Potentially symptomatic of many
hundreds of clinical conditions from diabetes to
nutritional deficiency and depression, tiredness
merits a prompt visit to the doctor if it arrived
out of the blue, has no obvious cause, or has
been unremitting for more than two weeks.
However, if you are not potentially unwell but
merely need to build up your energy levels, the
following essences can be fast-acting catalysts.
If none fits your bill, consider one of the
excellent general combinations such as Life
Force, Dynamis, or Essence of Energy.

Oak *(UK)*

— INDICATIONS

battling on mindlessly when totally exhausted
normally huge reserves of endurance and patience are depleted
continuing only through a strong sense of duty
refusing to rest, or admit weakness
usually a reliable linchpin, you're depressed by chronic overwork

+ EFFECTS

restores ability to rest
helps you become more flexible
reduces inner pressure to "go on, no matter what"
brings new vitality to heart and soul
promotes renewed energy, courage, and persistence

As well as the indications above, Oak is great for anyone who needs extra energy, courage, and perseverance under stress — say, when they are on a challenging trek, or for women in the latter stages of labor. It is often used to support recovery after a long illness, or when your reserves have been depleted by long-term stressful or demanding circumstances. Also consider Hornbeam, a tonic for that gray "Monday morning" feeling where the weariness is real enough but originates in the mind. For the "I'm so tired, I could cry" sense of utter physical and mental fatigue, try Olive.

Pyatã <small>(BRA)</small>

— INDICATIONS

you're facing major challenges, but are tired out
you're uninterested in life and depressed
you're giving up on projects
"courage batteries" are low; you would prefer everyone to leave you alone
for men experiencing erectile difficulties
you feel apathetic
your immunity is low, or you are convalescent
you lack appetite

+ EFFECTS

promotes recovery of willpower and persistence
facilitates the return of your vital force
stimulates self-preservation
combats depression/melancholy

Pyatã may stimulate your creativity, enthusiasm for life, and sexuality — all of which are closely linked, and among the first things to be affected by exhaustion. This essence is often used to enhance the libido and sheer enjoyment of sex, as well as for fertility issues and potency problems. When it works to help lighten your mood and raise your spirits, you will start to feel as if you have far more energy. Feeling down is very draining and tiring — feeling "up" has the opposite effect.

Welsh Poppy (UK)

— INDICATIONS

you've lost your old fire and inspiration

find yourself daydreaming too much

usually have plenty of energy, but it's gone

become sidetracked

previous goals have no meaning

you may fear it's due to others' negative influence and blame them for the
way you feel

+ EFFECTS

restores energy

renews inspiration

brings a new perspective to existing issues

This essence helps you realize when the problem isn't so much lack of
energy as that when old goals are seen in a new light they tend to lose
their attraction. Welsh Poppy helps show you your new path instead.
Then, when you are on the right track, your spirit is once again aligned
with what you are doing and you will feel more inspired, genuinely
committed, enthusiastic — and therefore more energetic as well.

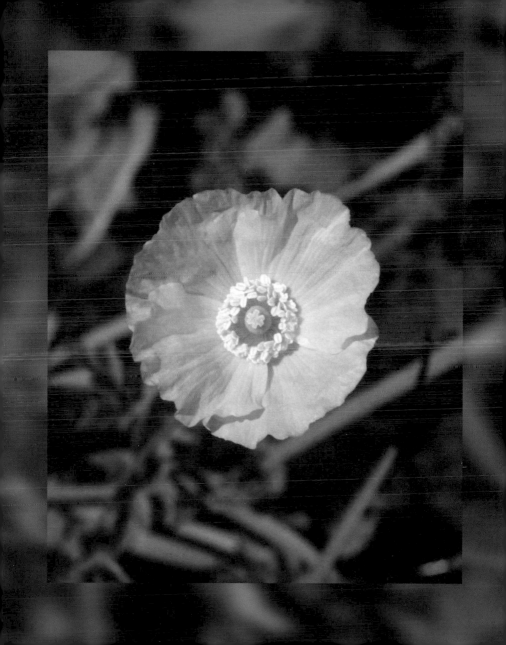

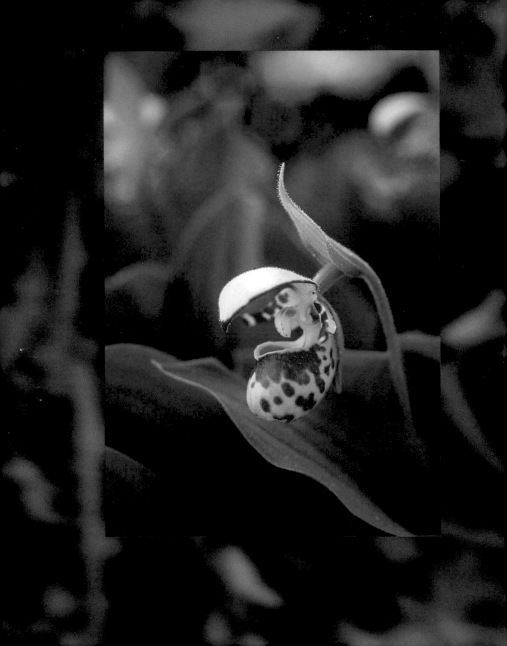

Lady's Slipper (ALASKA)

— INDICATIONS
resistance to receiving healing energy from others
lack of sensitivity to your own needs and energy flow
uneven energy flow through your central nervous system
uneven energy flow through your chakra system

+ EFFECTS
acts as a catalyst for receiving healing energy
regulates energy flow through the chakras and central nervous system
opens you to being helped

If you are feeling tired and depleted, you might visit a therapist such as a healer or reflexologist. However, if for some reason your own system is unable to take on board the extra energy on offer, they may find it quite difficult to help you. Lady's Slipper can act as a gentle catalyst to help you become open to the healing that is available. The essence can also be taken before or after an appointment: it can be useful if both the healer/therapist and the client take it.

Pink Fountain Triggerplant

(Aus)

— INDICATIONS

feeling as if your energy is slowly draining away

denying your body's physical needs

extreme tiredness/lethargy, initially caused by a shock or trauma to your body (surgery, viral infection, convalescence)

inability to regain your strength

you cannot cope

you're experiencing a sense of falling apart

+ EFFECTS

acts as a restorative

invigorates and strengthens

revitalizes

This essence can help restore your vital force, vigor, and stability when you just *cannot* seem to get back on top of things following illness, injury, or prolonged effort. If you are really run down, it is also well worth making sure that your aura (see page 11) is strong and unbroken. Physical injury, to the head in particular, may cause a split in your aura around the injury site through which your energy can literally drain away — this is partly why many people report feeling so tired after concussion. For advice on protecting and strengthening your aura, see pages 213, 219.

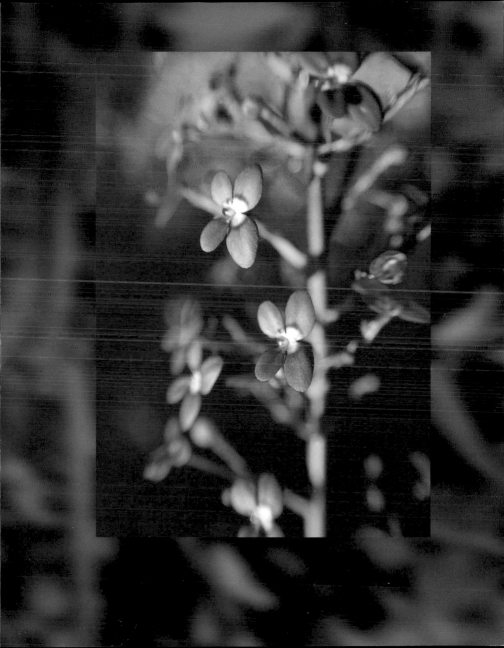

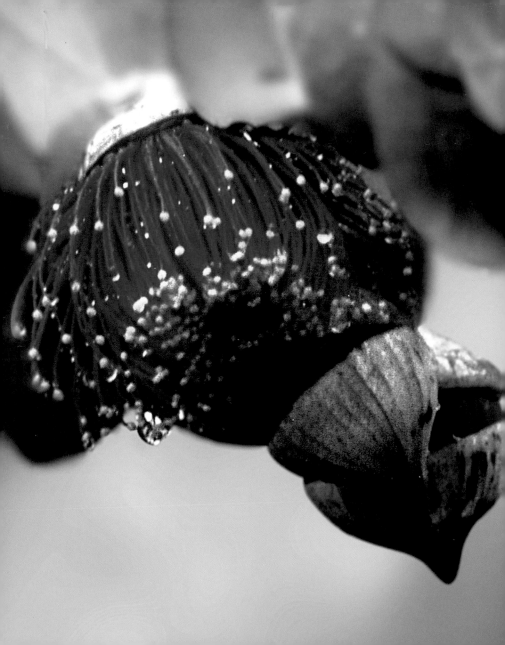

Macrocarpa (AUS)

— INDICATIONS

you're burned out
undergoing convalescence
exhaustion has set in
you've reached a difficult goal, but are now too tired to enjoy the
results/leisure afterward

+ EFFECTS

offers additional energy and vitality
produces renewed physical endurance
facilitates deeper sleep
restores your ability to rest

This is a popular urban remedy for city-dwellers and can be a good tonic for people who simply need a pick-me-up on a physical level. It can provide extra energy, as well as reinforcing the need for rest and sleep. Macrocarpa is also indicated when you have set yourself a challenging goal but find you are so exhausted after achieving it that you are in no state to enjoy your newfound leisure. If this is the case, combine this essence with Silver Princess, which is indicated for those who are feeling flat, aimless, and lacking in direction.

Vital Lift (UK)

— INDICATIONS

your energy is flagging but you need to stay on the case
it's important to keep going and finish something, but it's
beginning to look as if you may not make it
your attention is starting to waver

+ EFFECTS

acts immediately
can provide a rapid energy lift when urgently required
calms and aligns
keeps you going when you are fading
gives stamina for focused work

A fast-acting combination of five different orchid essences, Vital Lift is often chosen when you need energy *now*. The effect is closer to that of a good cup of tea than a strong coffee — it provides a centered "in the body" boost, unlike caffeine which can be too uncontrolled and robust for those who are sensitive. A good short-term remedy, this combination is not suitable for long-term use, nor for taking daily (or even frequently) in lieu of proper rest or recuperation.

Vital Spark (INDIA)

— INDICATIONS

feeling hopeless

depleted energy

tired all the time

experiencing weakness

recent shock, or fear

feeling stressed and fretful

+ EFFECTS

enhances vitality and life force

harmonizes your entire system

relaxes

rejuvenates

If you are tense, with your muscles rigid from sheer tiredness and the inability to sleep well, Vital Spark is a combination essence that helps you relax and let go, thereby allowing your body to realign itself and recharge its energy batteries. Consider also the Morning Glory (Himalayan variety) combination, which encourages sounder sleep, helping you get up and greet the day with enthusiasm. It can also be used to support you when you are trying to break an addictive habit like smoking, which saps your energy.

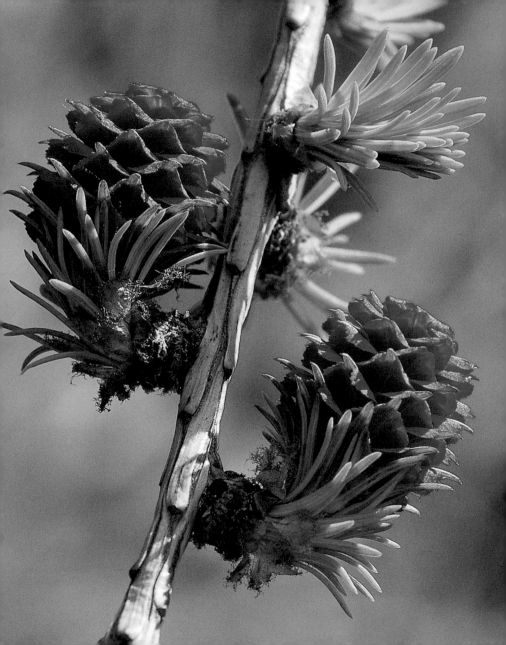

Confidence

Most of us probably feel we could do with a bit more confidence sometimes, but for some a real lack of it can make each day agony. True self-confidence is not arrogance — it's a quiet but unshakable belief in your own worth, and acceptance of yourself for who you are. That may take years to achieve, but once you have it, nothing — and no one — can ever take it away again. These essences can help you find this quality within yourself, but if none sounds as if it addresses the particular way you feel, try a good general combination such as Confid Essence, Self Esteem, or Strength instead.

LARCH

Larch (UK)

— INDICATIONS

you won't try, because you believe you will only fail

so convinced you can't do it that you feel useless

hesitant, passive

entirely capable, but lack confidence

may use illness as an excuse not to tackle something

false modesty due to lack of self-esteem

+ EFFECTS

removes "can't" from your vocabulary, although you
still assess things realistically

encourages you to persevere, even through setbacks

increases your willingness to have a go

replaces limiting concepts with confidence and real
belief in yourself

able to take a more relaxed view of life

A gentle can-do remedy, this essence is often used long-term to dissolve the self-limiting, negative programming that may beset Larch people — although you are just as capable as anyone else, and frequently more so. The essence helps you feel "I can do it, I will do it, I am doing it!" It is also helpful as a short-term focus remedy if you're nervous about an examination, driving test, or interview.

Inner Fire (UK)

— INDICATIONS

unable to end a situation that has become intolerable
have to draw a line in the sand *now*
lack of the fire and clarity you need to act
not enough power to stand your ground
fear of speaking out
feeling powerless

+ EFFECTS

facilitates powerful, decisive action
brings courage, clarity and fire energy
enhances your own inner power
encourages vision and discernment
helps you set firm boundaries

A combination of the energy of fire agate, fire pit, south red sandstone, and eagle's feather, this can be a very powerful essence. It allows you to say, "Right, that's it: enough is enough" in a way that insures your words are heard and respected. It is helpful for those raised in polite environments where it was not done to speak your mind, nor call a spade a spade. If you need to speak out firmly and clearly, or to draw clear boundaries after a period of having been taken advantage of or discounted in some way, Inner Fire can be a potent catalyst.

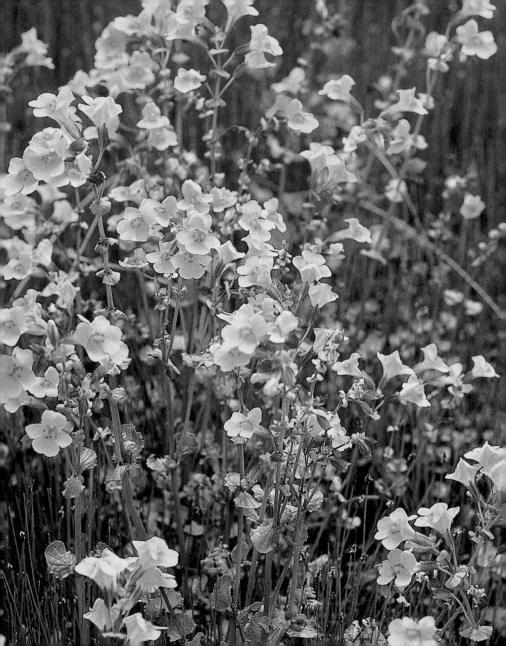

Monkey Flower (UK)

— INDICATIONS

giving away your power
on the defensive, yet over-apologetic
fearful of making another person angry
worried about being bullied
difficulty saying "No"
timid and nervous
fearful of disapproval, blame, criticism, ridicule, humiliation

+ EFFECTS

encourages you to stand in your power
enables you to act from strong inner convictions
helps you set clear boundaries
promotes boldness and assertiveness

Sometimes we are reluctant to be fully in our power for fear of
recriminations from other people or because we believe strength and
assertiveness are egotistical — which they aren't, anymore than standing
up for yourself when necessary could be called pushy. Monkey Flower
helps you find both your inner guidance and the strength and courage to
act upon it. It also fosters self-assurance, and a new fearlessness in
accepting feedback from others with equanimity.

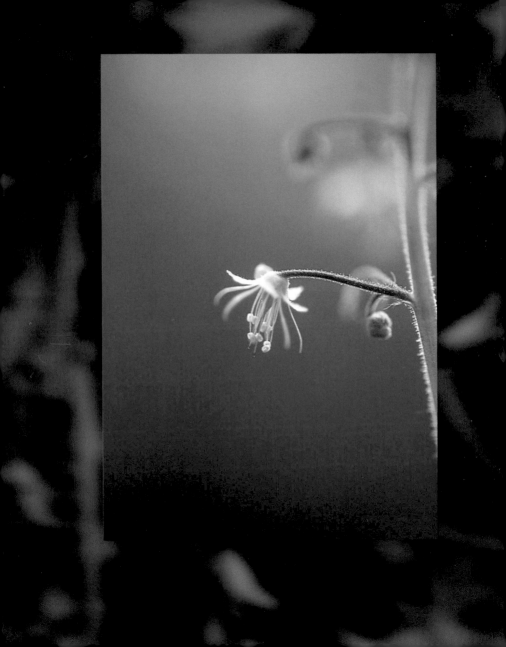

Lace Flower (ALASKA)

— INDICATIONS

feeling insignificant
victim of cultural bias or racial prejudice
experiencing sexual discrimination
suffering the negative effects of favoritism
low self-esteem

+ EFFECTS

brings knowledge of your own inner worth
enhances your ability to express your own unique talents
promotes healthy self-esteem
helps you understand and value your own role

This is a great essence for anyone who may be feeling a bit insignificant because they work within the home, or are based in a small town or out-of-the-way place. Lace Flower can remind everyone that no matter where you are, if you do whatever you can with love and awareness, this radiates outward and affects people around you in a powerfully positive way. It can also help show you that this in itself is really something, and matters just as much as the work of those who are more at the center of things or in the public eye.

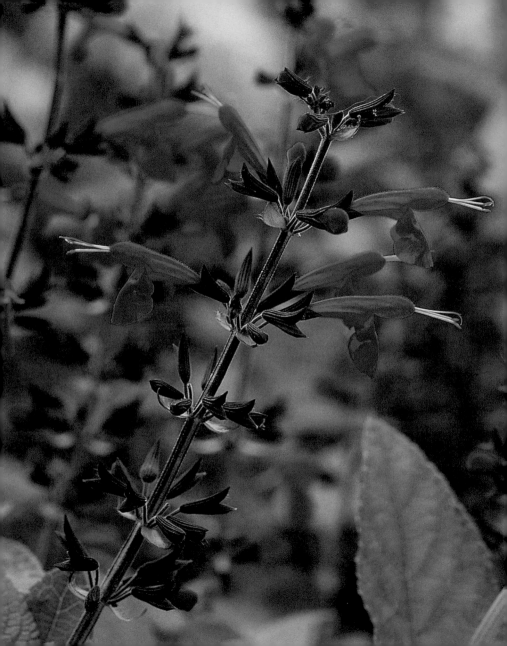

Salvia (USA)

— INDICATIONS

feeling overly self-conscious about your appearance
spending heavily on clothes, makeup, and beauty treatments
may develop anorexia
may become drug-dependent
lacking self-esteem

+ EFFECTS

helps you change your self-image for the better
brings sheer joy
encourages you to feel happy with the way you look
increases self-confidence

Salvia supports and encourages those who do not feel good about the way they look. This may range from an overconcern with minor defects that other people don't even perceive as such — a nose that its owner feels is too big, for example — to full-blown dysmorphophobia (common in anorexia) in which the sufferer cannot help seeing their own body as other than it is. This essence supports your new image, and your own body will complete the healing.

Mountain Lion (USA)

— INDICATIONS

worrying about what others may think

emotional weakness

not strong physically

lack of confidence

over-assertiveness

tendency to be "in people's faces"

+ EFFECTS

helps you stay true to yourself, despite what others may think

promotes courage and strength in challenging times

enables you to walk your talk

increases your ability to speak up for yourself

enhances self-assertion

Mountain Lion helps provide the courage you need to move through your fears. It also balances gentleness with the strength inside you, so can be helpful if you find you tend to come on too strong. This essence is useful if you are starting new projects because it can offer you powerful support in manifesting your dreams and visions. Consider also the Supreme Confidence combination (Mountain Lion, Bumblebee — and Cheetah, which can trigger swiftness, energy and a jump-start), a mixture that can offer valuable support to any new undertaking.

Five Corners (AUS)

— INDICATIONS
"crushed-in" personality
a need to keep apologizing for yourself
tendency to wear concealing clothing, and dull colors so as
not to draw attention
inability to feel good about yourself
self-sabotage

+ EFFECTS
enhances self-esteem
encourages love and acceptance of both yourself and your own body
helps you celebrate your own beauty
allows you to appreciate yourself in all ways
increases vitality

Have you ever had a relationship with someone who didn't really love themselves — and couldn't seem to accept your love either? This is a common pattern for people with low self-esteem, but Five Corners can encourage the release of negative, unhelpful beliefs and allow someone to blossom into the terrific person they really are. This essence can be very useful for adults, but is also important for any children and teenagers whose sense of self-worth is fragile.

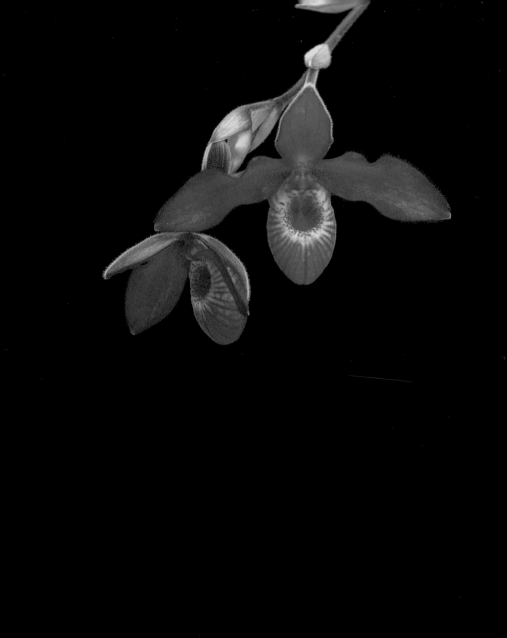

Andean Fire (UK)

— INDICATIONS

facing a huge physical challenge
overwhelmed by the suffering all around you
have been involved in a major disaster
for victims of torture
for those who have suffered greatly

+ EFFECTS

courage when you are afraid
helps you regain a sense of life purpose
ability to carry on through dark times
enables you to dare to make a leap

Its makers say that another name for this essence could be Resurrecting Courage and Purpose, for that is what it does for those who have faced severe challenges. Andean Fire can help those who have experienced religious or ethnic cleansing or persecution; or who have been caught up in natural disasters such as earthquakes and flooding where they saw great suffering and devastation; or who are survivors of oppressive political regimes. This remedy has also been used successfully for young children who need a one-off boost of courage, perhaps when they are afraid to meet a physical challenge but want to try anyway — such as attempting abseiling when they are afraid of heights.

Yellow Cone Flower (AUSTRALIA)

— INDICATIONS

needing to be validated by others because you feel inferior

craving social acceptance from your peer group

being used by others

feeling sad or depressed because you are being taken for granted

not recognizing your own value, thereby setting yourself
up for lack of respect

doing things for others because you need their recognition

+ EFFECTS

encourages you to recognize your own worth

brings inner confidence and contentment

helps you feel happier

This essence encourages the realization that the first and most important opinion is the one that you have about yourself. It helps create an inner sense of "Yes, I *am* OK." This can then dissolve the need for a recognition rating and validation from others, release you from needing or seeking their approval, and increase your confidence and self-esteem to healthy levels.

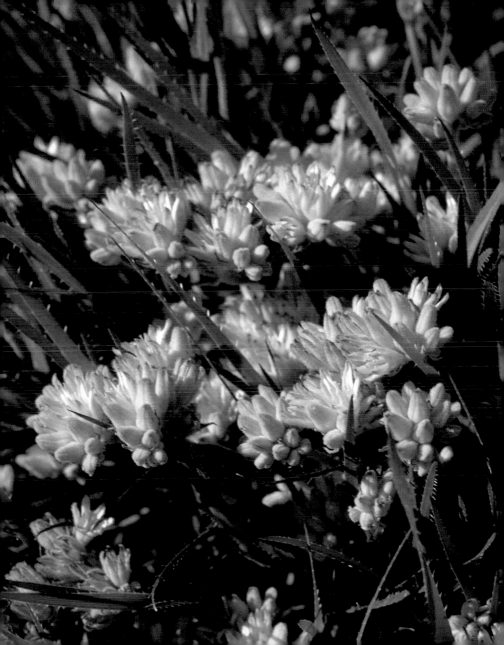

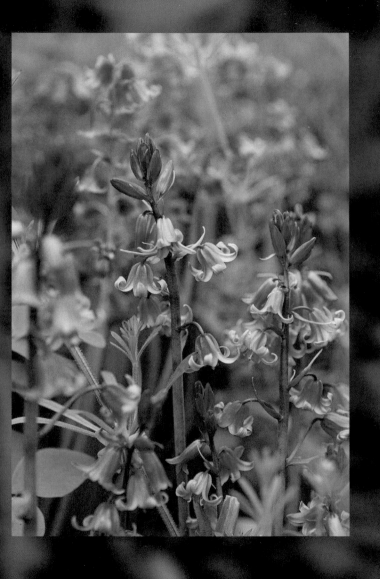

Bluebell (CAN)

— INDICATIONS

afraid of being ridiculed
anxious about being noticed at all
fearful of being punished
worried about being judged
troubled by shyness
autistic spectrum disorders

+ EFFECTS

helps you release old programs and engage in what really fulfills you
brings the courage to follow your vision of who you are
boosts low energy, combats fatigue
promotes easier breathing during panic or anxiety attacks
alleviates fear of self-expression and "being seen"

As children, we learn to behave in ways for which we are rewarded; we carry these memories into our adult lives at a cellular level, where they may stifle our ability to align ourselves with what we would really like to do, and can erode our confidence or ability to express ourselves freely. At an esoteric level, Bluebell supports the throat chakra (see pages 9–11); it is also often given for speech difficulties that have an emotional cause and for autistic spectrum disorders like Asperger's syndrome. Bluebell can also help combat shyness.

Oxalis *(S AF)*

— INDICATIONS

appearing to be self-important, but underneath burdened by
an inferiority complex
projecting a superior attitude to others
overbearing
struggling with dislike of self, even self-hatred
masking the above with an arrogant manner

+ EFFECTS

helps you set aside your armor
encourages development of your sense of self-worth
enhances your awareness of everyone's importance as part of the whole
brings humility

Oxalis is for those who mask an inferiority complex, a dislike (even hatred) of themselves, and the lack of confidence this brings, beneath an arrogant manner and self-important exterior. This essence helps you set aside the armor of superiority you have built around yourself for protection, and stimulates an appreciation of every single person's importance as a part of the whole. This makes it far easier for someone to love and respect themselves, enabling true self-confidence to blossom and grow.

Oyamã (BRA)

— INDICATIONS

lack of confidence, which leads you to wear social masks and
put on false personae
self-doubt and low self-esteem
anxiety, fear
deep sadness that refuses to lift
feeling of depression

+ EFFECTS

boosts assertiveness
enhances your ability to say "No"
brings confidence, and the vitality to project it
helps you toward self-acceptance and liking yourself
encourages strong conviction

The source of this remedy offers vivid clues to how it can help. Oyamã
is made from the flower of the cacao tree, and though it is a small,
vulnerable blossom, from it comes the powerful fruit that has given
the world chocolate, a substance that has comforted, energized, and
given pleasure to billions of people. This ability to transform something
small and fragile into a substance of great strength is contained within
Oyamã essence.

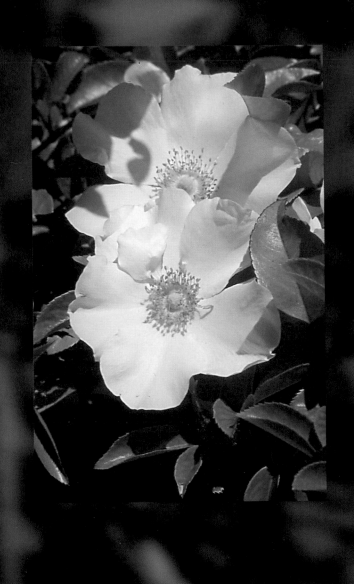

Joy

Joy's unique mixture of gladness, delight, and sheer ebullience lights up life. Lack of it may manifest anywhere along a wide spectrum of emotions, from feeling merely flat through to moderate depression, all the way to deep grief and distress. Some of the essences in this chapter can help lift your spirits and rekindle real exuberance and love of life; others can support people through profound unhappiness. Good combinations to try include Summer Solstice and Party Time, for uplift and fun — especially dancing and singing.

DOG ROSE

Dog Rose (S Af)

— INDICATIONS
grief that's denied, or not expressed
lacking the skills to speak your pain
old distress that is affecting the present
your aura has contracted, or shrunk, against further hurt

+ EFFECTS
helps you give voice to repressed grief, and there is magic in the telling
makes it easier to acknowledge your distress
encourages integration — and acceptance — of your pain

This South African Dog Rose essence (there are others from other countries, which have different qualities) can be especially helpful for children who are suppressing their emotions, or who find it difficult to say that they are hurt and talk about how they feel. In fact, it can be very helpful for anyone, of any age, who finds it hard to put their feelings into words, or who lacks the skills to express their pain. This type of Dog Rose essence supports the throat chakra, the energy center that governs communication skills — both speaking and listening — allowing the expression of deep emotions to flow more easily, and helping to release old distress which has become "stuck" either there or in the heart area.

Child Glow (USA)

— INDICATIONS
"every day feels the same"
gloom, despondency
heaviness of spirit
lack of sense of fun
not enjoying life one bit

+ EFFECTS
renews your sense of gaiety
allows you to delight in your existence
brings cheerfulness
promotes lightness of being

This ready-made combination is a good one for taking late in the afternoon or at the end of the day, when your spirits may be starting to drop — or to take four times a day for two to four weeks if you feel you are lacking cheerfulness and lightness in your life. Child Glow includes essence of Red Hollyhock (for faith and hope in life, with plenty of optimism and joy) and Lovage (for lightness, ease and fluidity of the body). Consider also Exaltation of Flowers, a combination of 56 essences.

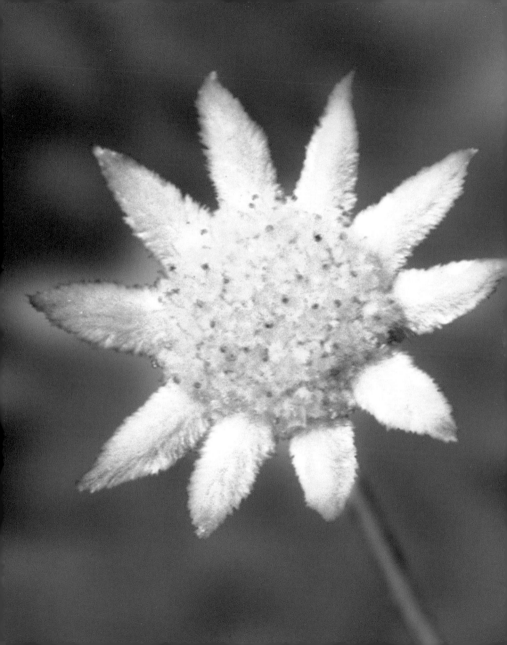

Little Flannel Flower (AUS)

— INDICATIONS
for overserious children
for children who are growing up too fast
for grim or "buttoned-up" adults
rigidity in outlook
lack of spontaneity

+ EFFECTS
allows you to have fun and feel carefree
brings joy
enhances playfulness
helps adults lose their inhibitions — and go play!
encourages spontaneity

This is the "lighten up" remedy. It is often used to help parents lose their inhibitions and have fun with their children — and with other adults. It also helps reconnect small children to their spirit guides, giving them back their awareness of the spiritual and angelic realms around them. Everyone has their own spirit guides and guardian angel to help and protect them (many "gut feelings" are actually gentle promptings from them) and most children are psychic or clairvoyant to some degree. Sadly, they are taught from an early age that it is not acceptable to mention such things ("Don't be silly") so they lose that important source of support.

Dianthus (USA)

— INDICATIONS
you suspect life just *isn't* going to work out
expectations, hopes, and desires are long forgotten
you feel no one cares about you
life is no fun anymore
you are apathetic, and not much interested in anything

+ EFFECTS
creates the feeling that each day is dawning brighter than the last
encourages a zest for life
allows a new joy to well up from within
promotes new ideas and increased creativity
stimulates new solutions to old issues or difficulties

This is an essence for those who are feeling "Oh, what's the point?" A
Dianthus personality is also often withdrawn and anemic, and therapists
note that people who need Dianthus frequently seem to have problems
with their spleen or pancreas, and are more likely to be struggling with
an eating disorder as well. This essence may help restore your zest for
living and a healthy, positive attitude.

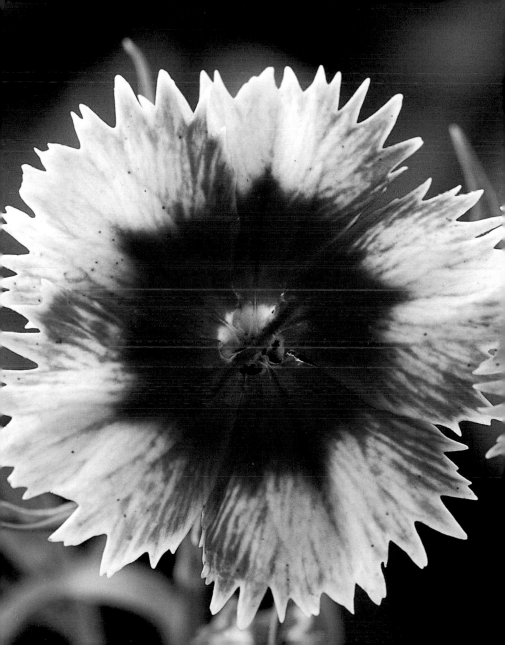

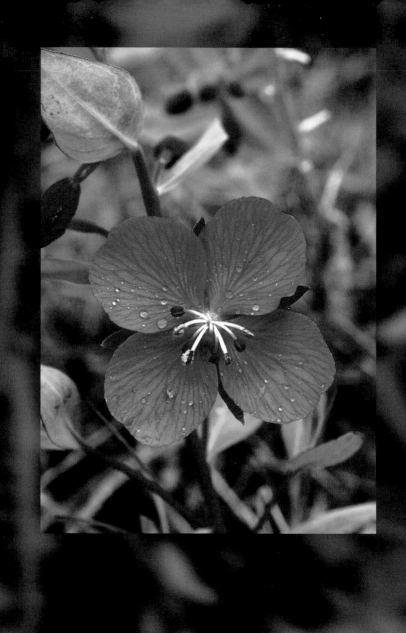

River Beauty (ALASKA)

— INDICATIONS

physical tightness/tension from unexpressed grief

shock after an accident, catastrophe, or loss

cannot regain your balance after traumatic events

difficulty letting go of emotional attachments to the past

emotional or sexual abuse

+ EFFECTS

releases physical tension resulting from unexpressed sadness

soothes traumatic effects of losing a loved one, relationship, or job

invites you to see adverse events as potential for growth and cleansing

supports emotional recovery

helps you get back your balance

This essence is for those struggling with overwhelming negative emotions. Perhaps you have experienced a "washing away" of a relationship or job; maybe there has been tragedy in your family or for a close friend. Floods are symbolic of great cleansing and radical change, and just as the River Beauty plant renews land after floods, its essence helps support and rebalance people after sudden dramatic events. Like a deluge of flood water, these events can literally sweep away the old to make way for new growth and eventual joyful transformation.

Jumping Child (Bra)

— INDICATIONS

stagnation

indolence, laziness

depression, discouragement, pessimism

difficulty in expressing your feelings

shyness, loneliness

difficulty in having fun, overly serious

+ EFFECTS

helps you feel happy

encourages spontaneity, and joy in living for the moment

increases vivacity, and enhances your sense of humor

promotes enthusiasm for life

stimulates self-expression, and vitality in speech

The first law of both physics and spiritual teaching is that energy can be neither created nor destroyed, merely changed from one form into another. And that is what this essence appears to do — transmute negative energy into positive energy. Jumping Child is made from a mushroom, and fungi have always been used to do this at the physical level: for example, composting organic waste into good garden fertilizer. This essence can also be used to support people who are timid, or who are feeling depressed or sad.

Hummingbird (USA)

— INDICATIONS

prevented from feeling joy by old emotional baggage
unresolved issues are holding you back
for those who've lost their sense of being *alive*
for anyone who needs to lighten up

+ EFFECTS

brings pure joy
offers uplifting support for those facing unresolved past issues
helps you celebrate being alive
encourages you to loosen up
enhances your ability to fool around and have fun

Hummingbird assists with the gentle purification and cleansing away of emotional residue, so it can be helpful if you have issues that need to be resolved before you are free to experience true joy. You can also try spraying the essence around a room to lighten a leaden atmosphere or lift people's spirits. It has often been used successfully in such situations when people are thoroughly fed up, to encourage relaxation and laughter.

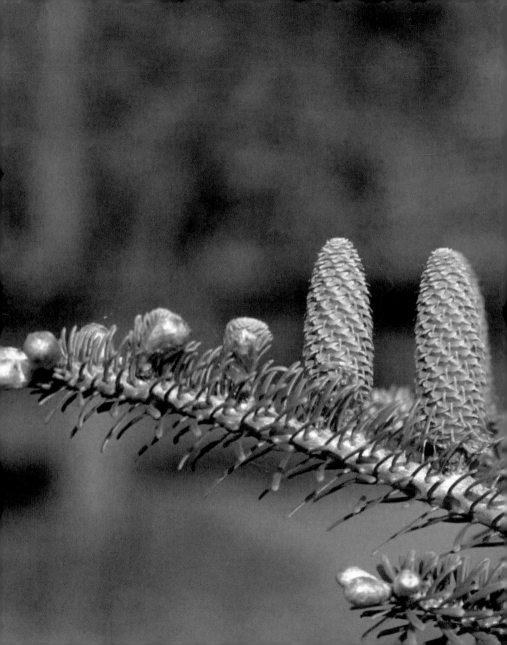

Arizona Fir (UK)

— INDICATIONS

assuming it isn't properly spiritual to delight in life

feeling there's something unsuitable in being joyful

believing that time on earth, since it's a learning experience, ought be hard

overascetic: a strong belief in "the path of suffering"

inability to enjoy or celebrate your existence

rigidity in outlook

+ EFFECTS

encourages you to live a spiritual life joyfully

helps you realize that spirituality and joy/happiness/
celebration aren't mutually exclusive

helps you open up

energizes the heart chakra (the center of love and emotion)

All too often, people may see spirituality as a rather grim and earnest business and become overserious about it all. This essence can stimulate a sense of freedom and joy, helping people loosen up and understand that earthly pleasures (like eating, drinking, dancing and laughing, having fun, and delighting in life) are essential to spiritual wellbeing, too, and part of a healthy balance in life. Arizona Fir encourages you to love and celebrate life — and also to love yourself.

Purple Crocus (CAN)

— INDICATIONS

grief and bereavement

deep sadness

turning your distress inward

feeling unable to mourn in your own way

your response to bereavement is rigidly dictated by your own culture

+ EFFECTS

helps you feel the true nature of your loss, and respond exactly
as you need to

encourages you to experience grief without resisting it

allows you to let go of the tension and heaviness of loss

This essence can be especially helpful for those who turn the force of their distress in upon themselves, rather than letting it out. Women are more likely to do this than men, and it is a process that has the potential to create life-threatening disease (see pages 9–11). Purple Crocus also helps reassure you that, regardless of what other, well-meaning people may say, when you are bereaved or saddened there is no "correct" way to mourn — only your own way, and this is the right way for you.

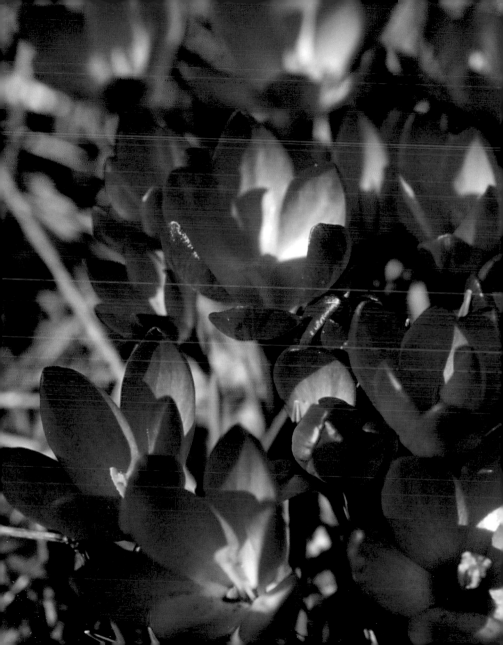

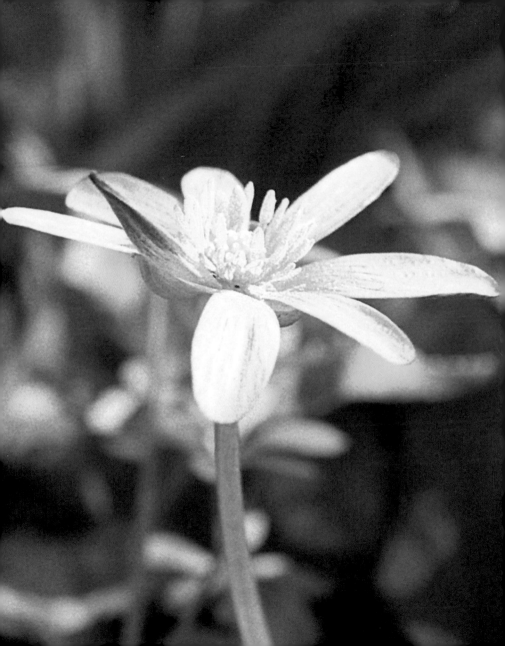

Mood lifters

Fed up? Worried and upset? Angry, or just plain
irritable? Then this is the chapter for you. It
looks at some of the most effective essences to
help lift your spirits and encourage a truly
positive, optimistic spin on life when it seems
to be going in only one direction: down (or
possibly flat) to match your mood. These
essences are about seeing the glass as half full
rather than half empty, and feeling that you do
deserve good things to happen to you —
therefore attracting them. They are also about
restoring genuine pleasure in living, taking off
the dark glasses, and knowing you have every
right to go after, and receive, all that you need.

Celandine (UK)

— INDICATIONS

gloomy, seeing the downside of everything
grumpy, negative, disgruntled, discontented
nit-picking, complaining
spreading gloom/bad news in conversation
world-weary, cynical

+ EFFECTS

helps renew your sense of appreciation and wonder
encourages renewed joy and delight
highlights the beauty and goodness in life
uplifting

This is the "taking off your dark glasses" remedy, a good one for getting you out of the habit of looking negatively at the world or at others. It can be very helpful for those times when you seem always to be looking for the worst, or for what's not right. Celandine shows you that you do have a choice about how you perceive things, and helps you focus on the good in your life or in the world: to see that glass as half full, rather than half empty.

Celebração! <small>(BRA)</small>

— INDICATIONS
flying around, always trying to find the answers outside yourself
lacking confidence, feeling helpless and/or submissive
cannot take pleasure in living
vulnerable, lonely, isolated
feeling dull, lacking in stimulation
tendency to complain

+ EFFECTS
calms a hyperactive, searching mind
helps you see life as a gift and an opportunity for self-development
enhances self-confidence, which lightens low mood
encourages you to take pleasure in your work
enables you to celebrate the sheer joy of living
"brings in light," allowing recognition of your own internal wisdom

A good essence for helping restore sheer love of life, joy, and self-confidence, Celebração! also encourages the realization that you already have the wisdom inside to find the answers you've been looking for all this time. It may also be helpful if you feel you tend to be overly drawn to gurus and other strong or forceful characters who seem to have all the answers, or if you sense that you may be in danger of becoming a workshop junkie in your quest for meaning.

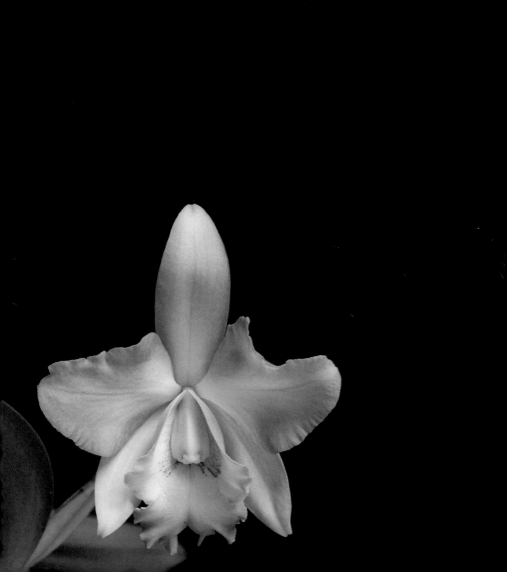

Angelic Canopy (UK)

— INDICATIONS

upset by an external event or disaster

in despair

experiencing grief

feeling tension and fear

for those who have lost hope

+ EFFECTS

brings nurturing support to those despairing or grieving

releases tension built from the fight/flight response to

danger and uncertainty

increases your sense of security

helps you realign your life values

A hybrid of the Laeliocattleya and Angel Love orchids, this essence was made nine days after 9/11 in response to the feelings of shock, insecurity, and distress ricocheting around much of the world at that time. It supports people in times of event-driven disaster, whether it be a terrorist attack, a major environmental crisis, or a negative but more localized event like the suspicious disappearance of a young child. Angelic Canopy is good for turbulent and unsettling times, or for living in a political and social climate of "feeling unsafe." It is also often used for space clearing in the home, office, or public spaces, and for cleansing crystals, too.

Red Hollyhock (USA)

— INDICATIONS

unhappy or uncomfortable with what you are doing
feeling unable to do something you need to do
depressed, sad
lacking in joy
experiencing loss of faith and hope

+ EFFECTS

brings the renewed energy that comes from aligning your
spirit to what you are doing
encourages you to tackle any project with enthusiasm
enhances your ability to be good-humored about everything
stimulates joy and optimism
restores faith and hope in life

This essence can be used for just a day to help adjust a temporary mood
— perhaps if a daunting task like compiling your tax return is looming
— as well as for the longer term. Helpful for invalids, it can also be taken
toward the end of demanding periods of medical treatment, such as anti-
cancer therapy or a series of operations. Red Hollyhock is an energy
booster, too, because it is thought to release any energy previously tied up
with depression and despair.

Otter (USA)

— INDICATIONS

need to stand back from a troubling situation but can't
chronically worried
overwhelmed by a situation or events
feeling down, depressed

+ EFFECTS

enables you not to take life too seriously
helps you worry less
allows you to step outside an upsetting situation to
reduce its emotional charge
brings in humor, laughter, and playfulness
encourages sheer delight in being alive

In addition to the indications above, Otter is appropriate for those who need to learn that life is not meant to be so difficult. It can also be a great support for children who are recovering from trauma, such as their parents' divorce. Besides encouraging play and joy, this essence helps you give some vital distance to troubling situations that would otherwise drain your energies, cease constant (sometimes pathological) worrying, and no longer feel overwhelmed by challenges. From a spiritual point of view, surrounding yourself with negative (worry) thoughts tends to attract more of the same, but fortunately the reverse is also true.

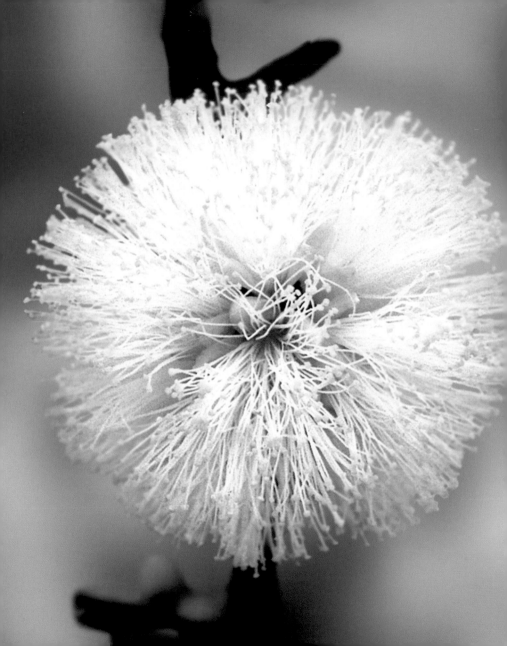

Sunshine Wattle *(AUS)*

— INDICATIONS

fully expecting a bleak or struggle-filled future
don't believe things will get any better
full of pessimism
a sense of hopelessness

+ EFFECTS

promotes a feeling of joyous expectation
stimulates optimism
helps you really look forward to the future
encourages belief in the positive possibilities of tomorrow

Sunshine Wattle works to bring about positive change if you have had a difficult time in the past, and now cannot seem to help expecting a repetition of the bad things that happened before. It is good, too, when your situation is temporarily difficult, nothing seems to be working out for you, and it feels as if life is just one big struggle. This essence has also produced good results for people who were worrying about money and feeling that their financial position was getting worse; many of them found that once they got on with living and enjoying life, those money problems just seemed to resolve.

Wild Violet (AUS)

— INDICATIONS

can't find a good word to say about anyone
complaining attitude
running down everything and everyone
for older people who can't feel positive any more
fatalistic, negative, killjoy, pessimistic
apprehensive underneath
attitude prevents you from experiencing life

+ EFFECTS

encourages optimism
enhances positivity
provides a good balance between caution and courageous decisions
helps you trust new opportunities, despite the unknown outcome
invites you to embrace life again

Wild Violet is great for that "Life's a bitch, and then you die" feeling; but if you are also feeling misunderstood and sorry for yourself, One-Sided Bottlebrush might be better. This helps if you are carrying a heavy load but feel that no one understands or appreciates this, and if you can't put yourself in other people's shoes. One-Sided Bottlebrush is often given to encourage people to develop a more lighthearted attitude to hardship, and also to put them in touch with the burdens that others have to carry.

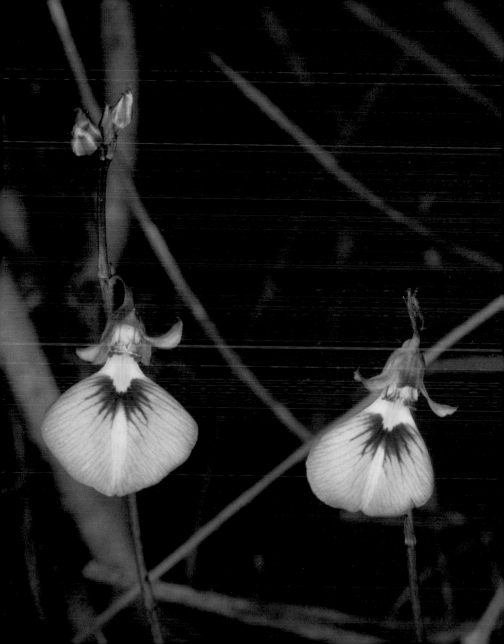

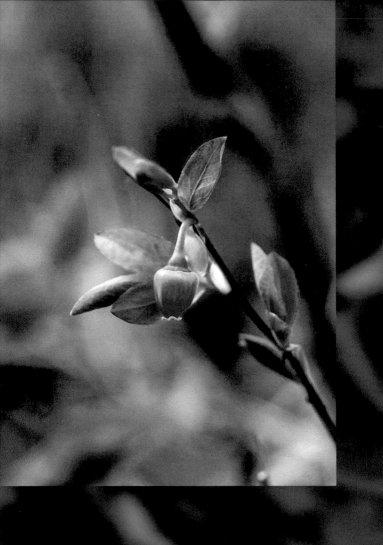

Blueberry Pollen (ALASKA)

— INDICATIONS

feeling you don't deserve good fortune

living in lack

expecting the worst

+ EFFECTS

encourages you to feel that you *do* deserve happiness

frees you from the feeling that you do not deserve good

fortune and abundance

boosts your self-esteem

One of the main spiritual laws is that "Energy Follows Thought." And one of the practical effects of this law is that if you are thinking something over and over, you tend to attract more of the same. Limiting or negative thoughts have powerful energy fields and a pulling power that reels in still more negativity and limitation, interfering with your ability to receive. Yet positive thoughts attract still more positivity. Blueberry Pollen essence helps release any deeply held beliefs that tell you that somehow you don't deserve to be happy or have what you need — leaving you free to attract what you desire (and more) in all its glory.

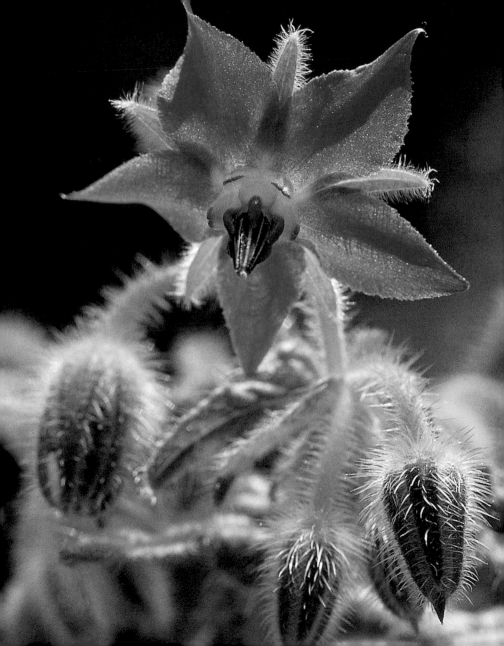

Women

Women are powerful, creative, nurturing, and astounding, despite having to deal with many demands on their energies (and challenges to their health and general equilibrium) that men do not. But because most women have their own lives to lead yet also have children, and because from puberty to the end of menopause they have to contend with constantly fluctuating hormone levels, they may need extra support at particular times: during adolescence, the fertile and child-rearing years, and when that fertility slows and ceases. Flower essences, perhaps the most deep-acting and feminine of all complementary therapies, are ideally equipped to offer special support to women. Good combinations can be effective too — consider Inner Female Essence, Serenity for Women, or Woman Essence.

BORAGE

Borage (NLD)

— INDICATIONS
you are pregnant, but feel no connection with your unborn baby
discouraged, downhearted
losing faith
experiencing problems becoming pregnant

+ EFFECTS
helps pregnant women to connect to the soul of their unborn child
strengthens the heart in difficult circumstances
prevents you from feeling discouraged by difficulties
brings joy and faith
may facilitate conception
supports women undergoing fertility treatment

Borage helps to connect pregnant women with the spirit of their unborn child — something many mothers find they do anyway. (Groundbreaking research in the 1980s by gynecologist Dr. David Cheek in San Francisco supports the reality of the telepathic connection between mothers and their unborn babies.) If you are pregnant, consider also Angelica, which can offer psychic protection for unborn babies. Some therapists who are also healers may ask a woman to hold a bottle of Borage essence over her thymus gland during a treatment, then take it as normal afterward.

Ruby-Kyanite 2 (EIRE)

— INDICATIONS

feeling second best to men

experiencing the need to be submissive/subjugated to men

being passive-aggressive to get your own way

feeling used sexually, but believing this is somehow permitted

+ EFFECTS

brings the knowledge — and belief — that men and women are equal

builds the confidence to show this in your behavior and choices

enables you to let go of any sexual or social patterns that do not serve you

This gem essence helps you let go of any unhelpful or disempowering patterns that do not support you, which you have taken on from your own mother and grandmother. These include automatic subservience, manipulation, negative expectations based on the past, not feeling good enough — all patterns that can be stamped into the emotional DNA and continue to replay generation after generation, blocking many women from coming into their true power and reclaiming their real place in the order of things. Until, that is, you are able to set those patterns aside once and for all.

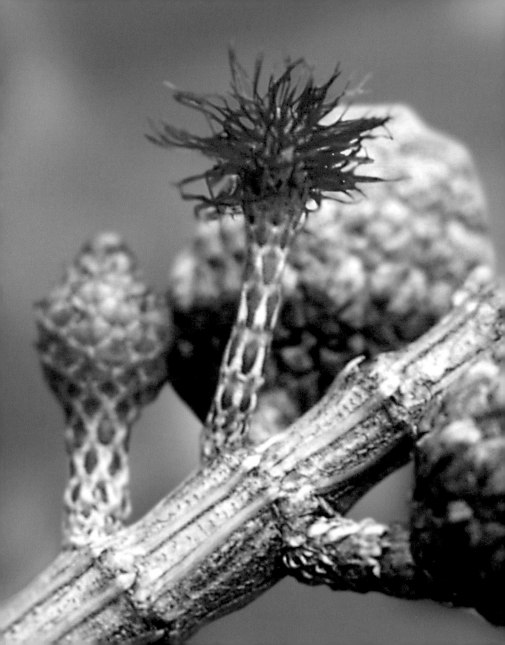

She Oak (AUS)

— INDICATIONS

premenstrual syndrome (PMS), including sore breasts and fluid retention
troublesome periods
negative side effects of the menopause
fertility problems, with or without an obvious cause

+ EFFECTS

improves hormonal balance
given to enhance fertility
helps regulate women's cycles
promotes hydration of the body
is used to encourage easier periods

For PMS with mood swings, therapists often combine it with Peach Flowered Tea-Tree. She Oak is offered as a gentle, safe alternative to HRT by many therapists — as is the Brazilian Embó Rudá — and also by a few progressive Australian, Brazilian, and Swiss gynecologists. A long-term, double-blind clinical trial is currently being carried out in Australia (results 2006) on She Oak's efficacy in fertility problems. This essence is often given for a wide variety of period difficulties, too, including heavy bleeding and painful cramps. It may also be used with Flannel Flower (see page 121) to help clear any past-life issues that, on a spiritual level, could be blocking your ability to conceive.

Candystick (CAN)

— INDICATIONS

miscarriage: trauma and distress

abortion: ambivalence, guilt, grief, trauma

problems concerning sexuality, or birth itself

anger, frustration

any invasive incident for the reproductive system, including surgery

injuries to the sacral area, or pelvic girdle (for women and men)

+ EFFECTS

in miscarriage: nurtures a willingness to honor the free will of
the unborn baby's soul

after abortion: helps you learn to live with, and honor, your choice

brings perspective

transforms anger and frustration

Candystick addresses the fact that, apart from physical trauma, both miscarriage and abortion may have other aspects to them for many woman. The distress of a pregnancy ending, or being ended, before term, can last for many years, even if it was the result of a free choice made by the woman herself. Also, if you visit an essence therapist knowing that you need something but without any clear idea of why you are there, Candystick may be prescribed, for it can support you in finding your soul's purpose.

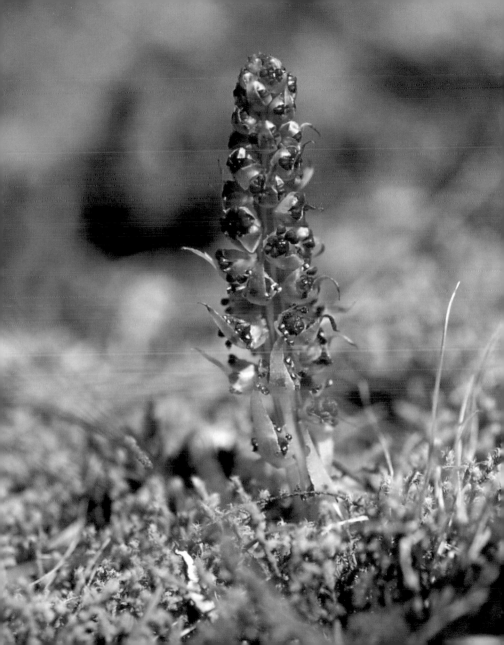

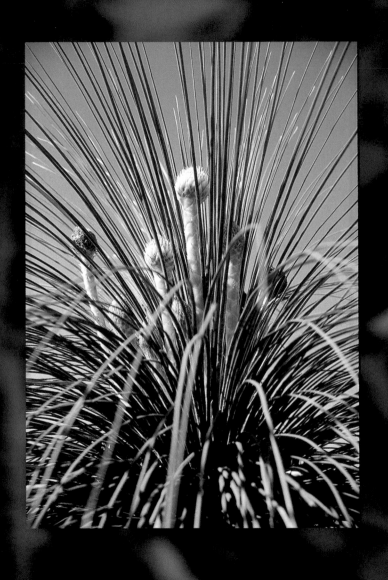

Goddess Grasstree (AUS)

— INDICATIONS

you're a first-time mother feeling alien to your new role

you have mothering issues

difficulty being patient

are unable to bring out your compassionate side

tend to resort to your emotions to deal with relationships

+ EFFECTS

develops your caring strength, which helps to bring out strength in those you look after, too

creates love and care that are not emotionally dependent

helps you become comfortable and balanced as a mother

This essence is especially for mothering issues. It can help you if you find you are using guilt to maintain control, have difficulty allowing independence in those you look after, or are unable to enjoy nurturing someone vulnerable in your care. It is also for balance, as it is a remedy that helps create a strength that is nurturing and caring, while bringing out the strength in the other person, too. It is often used for balancing period problems and female hormones as well.

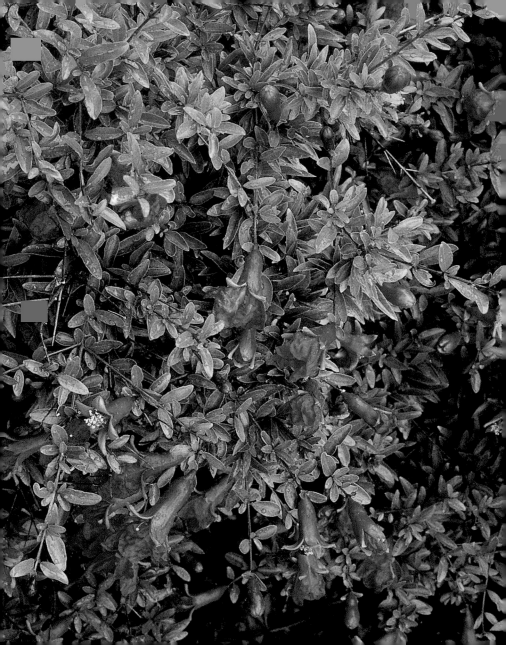

Pomegranate (S AF)

— INDICATIONS
demands of your career and home are out of balance
trying to be Superwoman
puberty, pregnancy, or menopause
sexual issues
problems conceiving
premenstrual syndrome (PMS)

+ EFFECTS
balances the male and female aspects of yourself
helps establish your identity as a woman
frees your female creativity
works for balance in times of hormonal change
encourages you to feel comfortable with your sexuality

"Feminine" energy, whether in a man or a woman, is enormously creative. This is one reason why many women in the middle months of pregnancy find they have a strong surge of artistic or "making things" energy, using it to write, paint, design, beautify, or construct. Pomegranate helps put people of both sexes in touch with this aspect of themselves. It can also be used to support you through puberty, pregnancy, menopause, or sexual issues — in fact, anything relating to the female procreative force.

Grove Sandwort (ALASKA)

— INDICATIONS

mother-and-child bond lacks warmth and vitality
you have difficulty nursing your baby
with several young children in the family, you feel overwhelmed
you feel unloved
you try to get your affection or nurturing inappropriately

+ EFFECTS

fosters a close, loving bond between mother and child
eases nursing problems for babies and their mothers
helps children feel supported and cared for, even when
their parents are away
allows the mother to feel supported when the father is away

This is a nurturing remedy (for both giving it to others, and for feeling it yourself) and also an important essence if you didn't have the love and care you needed or deserved when you were a child. Many try to make up for this (often unconsciously) by expecting their adult partners to provide it instead, but this is something that places a heavy burden on the other person and can be a major cause of repeated relationship failure.

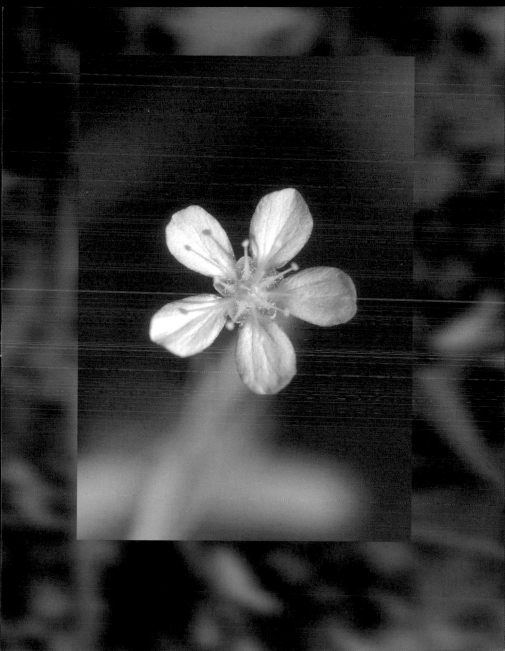

Heart Mother (UK)

— INDICATIONS

For mothers who:
overprotect their children, which disempowers them
need to stand back from their children, cut the apron strings
give too much to the family or others
are too hard on their children
do not offer them enough nurturing and support
had too little or too much mothering themselves
swing between self-denial and neediness

+ EFFECTS

getting your life back
not needing to help others in order to feel worthy
worrying less about those in your care

A combination of Cyclamen and clear quartz, Heart Mother embodies the balanced, archetypal mother inside us all: strong, gentle, and wise, a being who respects her own needs and nurtures without smothering. She is the mother who encourages her children to leave the safety of her arms so that they may explore life, growing in wisdom and experience. This essence is great if you are a supportive, loving mother but find you are overinvolved with your children's problems to the point of debilitating yourself, for it will help you give those issues some healthy distance.

Pre-Natal Heal (USA)

— INDICATIONS
worried or fearful about giving birth
feeling inadequate about your own mothering ability
old birth problems show up on "delivery anniversaries"

+ EFFECTS
helps you heal any fears or traumas about labour
allows you to visualize motherhood clearly and positively
encourages calmer, confident childbirth

This combination essence includes Catmint, Dogwood, Motherwort, Snow Queen Iris, and many others. It can be especially helpful for women who have had a difficult time in labor before, or who carry negative memories dating way back to their own birth, buried deep in their subconscious. These memories can be very strong: Psychotherapy regression studies comparing the memories of subjects under light hypnosis with their obstetric birth records (which they had never seen) show a remarkable factual correlation of events, including whether there was a difficult assisted delivery or if the baby became stuck in the birth canal. Pre-Natal Heal is also useful for physical problems stemming from birth trauma that show up in the reproductive tract, recurring on birth anniversaries — such as a uterus prolapse that appears yearly around the original delivery date.

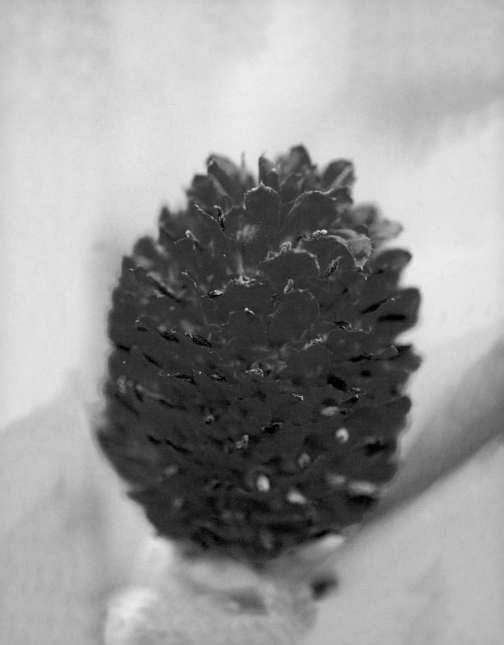

Men

Men have had to cope with a huge amount of change over the last 25 years, and more is on its way. Old role models are disappearing and traditional very male ways are increasingly less appropriate, yet there are few guidelines about new ways of being. All this comes at a time when both sexes need to balance the masculine and feminine sides of their natures, becoming complementary but equal partners while retaining their own sexual and social identities. It is time now for men to begin first to honor, then to integrate, the female aspects of themselves — understanding that they can be strong achievers while also treating others with compassion and gentleness. Essences can help with just that.

Bromelia 2 (BRA)

— INDICATIONS

uncertainty, embarrassment, or ambivalence over your own male sexuality

shame over your homosexuality

sexual repression

fear that your feelings and appetites may be inappropriate

tyranny, overdomination

repressed aggression

+ EFFECTS

helps you clarify your sexual identity

allows you to be in contact with your sexual instincts without fear

releases and integrates hidden emotions

enables you to be positive and comfortable about your

own sexual orientation

One underlying action of this essence is unification and balance — it encourages any more aggressive male energies (which can lean over into tyranny and domination) to be balanced by strong female forces. Both coexist naturally in the makeup of each sex anyway, just in different ratios. A clue to one of the ways this essence works lies in the plant's appearance — sharp aggressive leaves growing in clumps, with showy reddish and purple flowers — yet those leaves also retain water which quenches the thirst of small forest animals, and frogs take refuge there too.

Balga Blackboy (AUS)

— INDICATIONS

very goal-oriented

aggressive

overpowering, overly macho

for adolescents who have difficulty integrating their assertive new sexuality

too little masculine power, or too much

negative, dangerous, or destructive feelings

+ EFFECTS

helps you become calmly assertive and forthright

balances achievement with life-sustaining qualities

This essence is used to support the maturing and balancing out of everyone's male side, so from this point of view, it is a good essence for both men and women. It can help you know that it is possible to be both assertive and caring, and that in the times in which we are now living you no longer have to make a choice between one and the other. Balga Blackboy also encourages a more relaxed attitude to achieving the goals you have set yourself, so that you can be strongly focused without becoming either blinkered or obsessed.

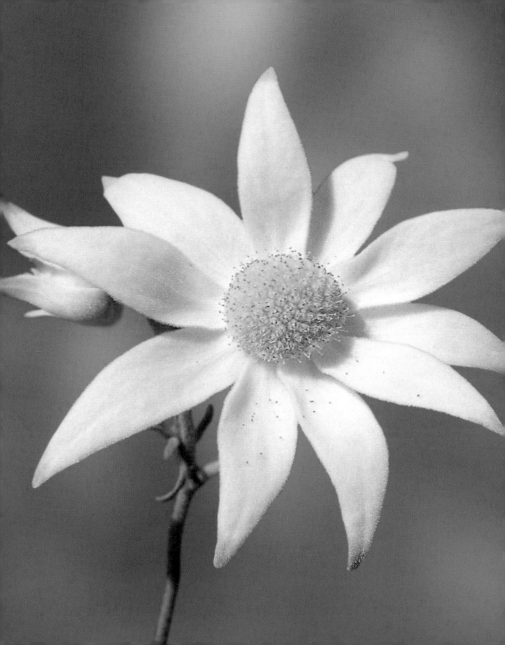

Flannel Flower (AUS)

— INDICATIONS

unable to say how you feel
uncomfortable about being touched
the idea of emotional intimacy makes you ill at ease
you have been physically attacked — mugged or assaulted
you have been sexually abused

+ EFFECTS

allows you to trust, and open up
releases your inhibitions about physical contact and being touched
enables you to express your feelings more easily
helps enjoyment of physical expression via movement, dancing, or sport
provides a healthy perception of personal space (your own or others')
encourages gentleness

Flannel Flower is the remedy for physical expression. It is especially helpful if you don't like to be touched but crave physical closeness and contact, or can't get close to others easily even though you long to — then, when you do, you feel your personal space has been invaded, so social contact and being in crowded places can be very uncomfortable. While it tends to be a male remedy, this essence can work equally well for women. Flannel Flower also encourages the establishment of firm emotional boundaries.

Azalea (S AF)

— INDICATIONS
difficulties with fathering
trouble bonding with your children
unaware of the importance of your role as a dad
rebelling against authority figures
overly obedient, or overawed by authority

+ EFFECTS
supports and develops your role as a father
helps you bond with your sons and daughters
fosters an appropriate reaction to authority
encourages teenage sons to come into their power

Appropriate for fathers of children of any age, Azalea is especially helpful for dads with teenage sons. As you feel the nature of your relationship change, it can help to work toward offering your sons a positive role model and showing them good "ways of being," while retaining healthy structure and boundaries. This essence is for sons, too, as they begin to grow into their own personal power and identity. It can also help someone develop a balanced, comfortable attitude toward authority — neither too confrontational nor overeager to please.

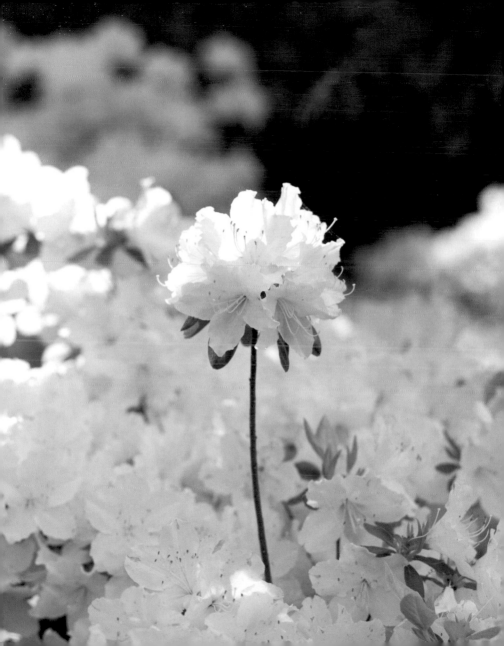

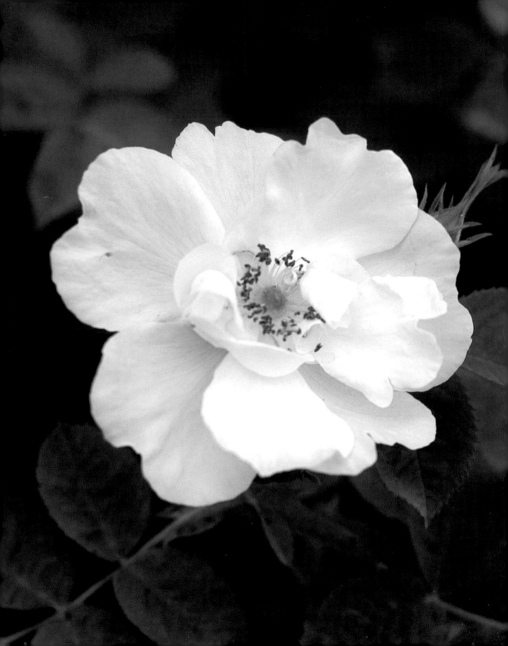

Rosa Alba (UK)

— INDICATIONS
overstrong drive for power and control
tendency to abuse your power
dictatorial, authoritarian, overbearing
proud, arrogant, stubborn
critical and judgmental
emotionally insecure
feeling inadequate, ineffective, impotent

+ EFFECTS
promotes leadership and the enlightened use of individual power
encourages you to speak from an inner authority
fosters determination and perseverance
helps develop strength, benevolence, and honor
heals the father/son principle

This essence is about letting go of the need to control, and it supports the correct use of power — for without love, power can easily be misused. Rosa Alba helps you find the strength and authority to walk your talk, and encourages you to let go of feelings of inadequacy or pride or any entrenched control patterns you have learned. It is useful for both men and women, but may be especially helpful to men. The remedy can also be used to support virility and potency.

Bumblebee *(USA)*

− INDICATIONS

always wanting to succeed at an ever higher level
seldom satisfied with your own achievements
lacking in confidence
discouraged by obstacles and limitations

+ EFFECTS

enables you to break through your apparent limitations
helps you achieve what once seemed impossible
encourages you to express your power and special gifts with confidence

This essence uses the special "energy" of the bumblebee only, for no creature is ever captured or hurt when an animal essence is made. Instead, all Wild Earth animal essences like this one are made by a special attunement ceremony in the wild. Bumblebee is for claiming your power as a strong and fully capable person. This essence nurtures strength, a feeling of invincibility, and supreme confidence in your abilities, supporting you in achieving what otherwise would have seemed completely out of your reach.

Sea Horse (CAN)

— INDICATIONS
rigid ideas as to how men and women are supposed to be

laziness

lack of vitality

+ EFFECTS
enhances physical performance

helps the lungs to take in more life force via the breath (prana)

accesses the "wild one" inside you

brings the knowledge that there is no loss of power in gentleness

enhances vitality and energy

Like all animal remedies, this one is made just from the unique energy of the sea horse without harming or even touching the animal itself. This is a remedy of choice for athletes and is also used to support male fertility. However, if you are seriously striving for sports excellence, whether at amateur or professional level, Surfgrass may be suggested, too, since therapists report that it strengthens the will and can help provide a "second wind."

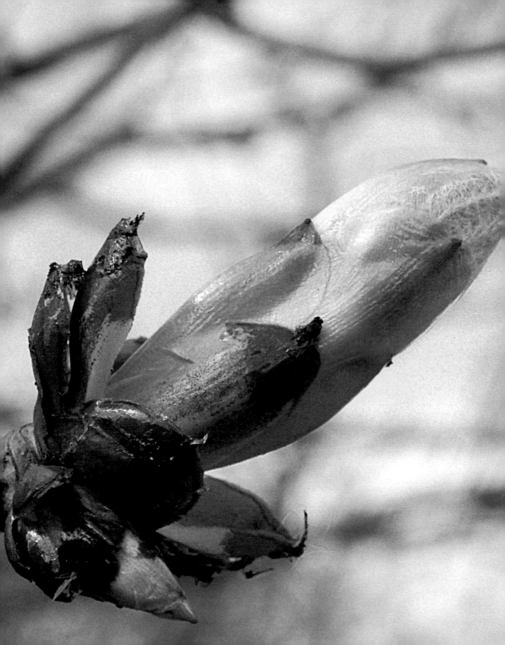

Sex

Sex can be one of the greatest pleasures there is, and being able to express sexuality joyously and freely is the right of every living being. The keys to a happy sex life (apart from available partners) include feeling comfortable with the physical side, having balanced sexual energies, and being able to connect emotionally and to both give and receive affection and love. When it comes to sexual difficulties, most seem to have their roots in a lack of self-esteem, embarrassment, difficulty in communicating, or an imbalance of sexual energy — all issues with which essences can help. Good general combination mixes that support sexuality as a whole include Love Life Plus for Men, Sexuality, Eros, and Make Love.

HORSE CHESTNUT LEAF BUD

Horse Chestnut Leaf Bud (UK)

— INDICATIONS

for women who:

like emotional/spiritual closeness with men, but uncomfortable about sex

are turned off by sex

dislike or fear men's sexual energy, and male bodies

for men who:

have experienced peer pressure/judgments of their sexuality/physique

don't feel good about their own sexuality or body

have been rejected before by partners on that basis

find enjoyment of their body is affected by cultural or religious attitudes

+ EFFECTS

for women:

encourages an attraction to, and real enjoyment of, good sex

restores their attraction to, and enjoyment of, male sexuality

for men:

brings a deep appreciation and understanding of own male sexual energy

inspires them to offer this maleness with love and tenderness

This remedy can be equally helpful for both men and women, allowing both sexes to feel good about their bodies, at home in them, and comfortable about sexuality — both their own and that of their partner.

Tufted Vetch (UK)

— INDICATIONS
difficulty relating to the opposite sex

guilt about sex

embarrassment over the act of sex or sexuality in general

lack of balance between your male and female sides

+ EFFECTS
encourages you to see sex as a natural part of living

helps you relate more easily to the opposite sex

allows you to feel joyful about your own sexuality

promotes a better balance of male–female within yourself

The human sex drive can be very strong but, like money and power, it is often used to manipulate or control others. This essence brings the two sides of your nature, male and female, into better balance, helping you to feel comfortable with and to honor your own sexuality and, therefore, that of others as well. Two combination essences, Yin and Yang, may also be indicated if you feel you need Tufted Vetch.

Wood Betony *(USA)*

— INDICATIONS

inappropriate sexual behavior
difficulty integrating love into your sexuality
overly focused on sex

+ EFFECTS

encourages you to be sensual
helps you develop a healthy relationship with sex
harmonizes the way you express your own sexuality
balances your flow of sexual energy

It is helpful to add Fox Mountain's Black-Eyed Susan essence (different from the Bush variety) if you suspect that inappropriate sexual behavior, or urges to behave in a particular way, are being caused by old abuse issues buried at a subconscious level. Be willing and ready to deal with these when they come up — if they do start to surface, you may want to consider therapy or appropriate support to help you through.

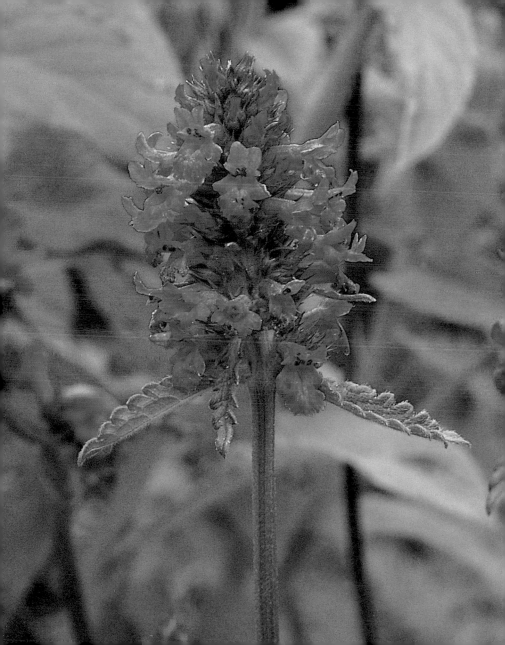

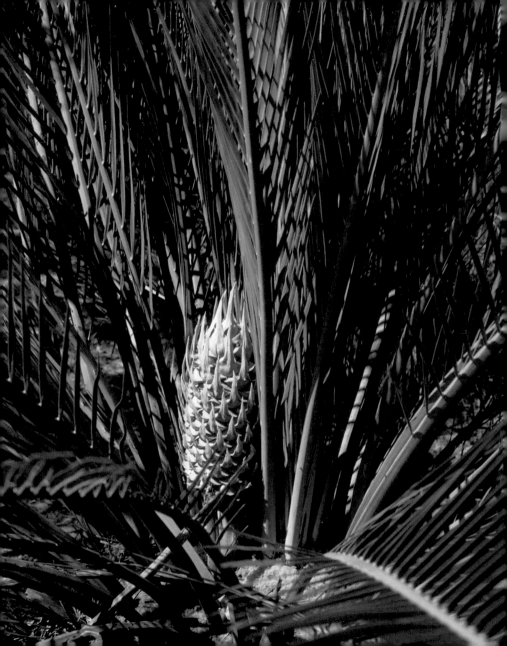

Macrozamia (Aus)

— INDICATIONS

continually attracting the wrong sort of person
sexual problems in general
overly focused on sex
frigidity or impotence
negative feelings about sex, inhibitions
low sexual self-esteem
difficulty trusting
sexual stereotyping

+ EFFECTS

balances the masculine and feminine sides within you
creates sexual wholeness
enables you to be comfortable and happy with love and sexuality

There are many reasons for negative (problem-causing) sexual imbalance, ranging from being around unhealthy imagery of sexuality when you were a child to distressing early sexual experiences. You may react to these by focusing too much on sex, by freezing up, or by perpetrating your negative feelings about sexuality by repeatedly attracting the "wrong" kind of partners, who do not make you happy. Macrozamia is a good all-round balancer and is used to help resolve sexual problems of most kinds, including those listed above.

Balsam (UK)

— INDICATIONS

unfulfilled desire
feeling unloved, unwanted, abandoned, rejected
fear of intimacy
coldness, frigidity, aloofness
dislike of physicality

+ EFFECTS

brings warmth, sensitivity, sensuality
helps you feel at home in your body
allows you to become comfortable with your sexuality
encourages you to celebrate your body
facilitates relationship bonding
enables you to nurture and nourish yourself, and others

When you do not feel at home in your body, perhaps because you feel out of place or ill at ease or are failing to nourish yourself, you may have difficulty relating to others, feel separate from them, or simply have a sense of being unloved. In these situations, Balsam can help you experience feelings of tenderness, warmth, and sensitivity toward yourself and others. It also strengthens mother/child warmth and bonding, especially if there has been separation, and is often used to support people who have experienced sexual abuse.

Heart of Tantra (INDIA)

— INDICATIONS

fear of love in sexual relationships

using sex for power

sexual aggression

rigid attitudes toward sexuality

+ EFFECTS

connects sex with love

encourages playfulness in sex

opens up sexual channels of communication

This essence helps create a bridge between the center of love and emotions (the heart chakra) and the center of sexuality and reproduction (the powerful sacral chakra, located — according to esoteric teachings — deep in the body between the pubis and navel). Instead of these two feelings and types of energy remaining separate — as "love" on one side and "sex" on the other, a division that exists for many, especially when they are quite young — Heart of Tantra encourages it to feel easy and natural for you to allow love, as well as sheer physical enjoyment, to be part of your sexual relationships with others.

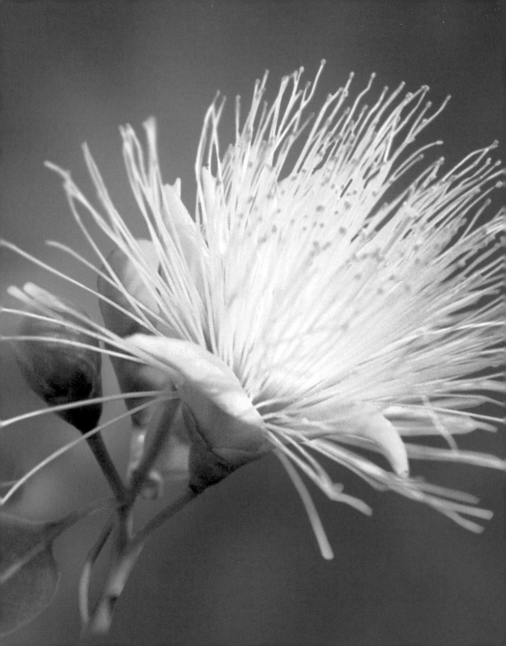

Billy Goat Plum (AUS)

− INDICATIONS
feelings of disgust or dislike about sex
disliking your own body or genitals
shame
difficulty enjoying sex
feeling defiled because of past assault or abuse

+ EFFECTS
encourages wholehearted sexual enjoyment
helps you feel comfortable with sex
brings joyful acceptance of your own physical body

This essence can be equally helpful for both men and women who feel distaste for the physicality of sex or sexuality, including dislike of the body's natural healthy secretions such as sweat or sexual juices. Billy Goat Plum is also used both topically and internally for rashes, including psoriasis and eczema, and is indicated as a bath or diluted wash for itchy or rash-based skin conditions anywhere on the body, if the disorder produces a sense of your body being somehow unclean. It may also be used for any feelings of self-disgust, not just those related to sex.

Basil (S AF)

— INDICATIONS

can't be sexually faithful, even when you try
promiscuous
into illicit or debasing sexual activity
fixated on/addicted to pornography
ruled by your genitals
physical gratification is the top priority

+ EFFECTS

balances and harmonizes sexual energies
can help those who wish to be faithful to one partner

In Western society, we are given mixed messages about sexuality, so
hypocrisy and secrecy around sexual attitudes are rife. Yet besides being
a potential source of great physical pleasure and a route to emotional
intimacy and love, sexual energy can also be a powerful spiritualizing
force and a tool for enlightenment. However, misunderstanding or
misusing it will hold you back on your path to spiritual development.
This essence helps you understand the "higher octave" of sexuality,
and supports you in becoming whole.

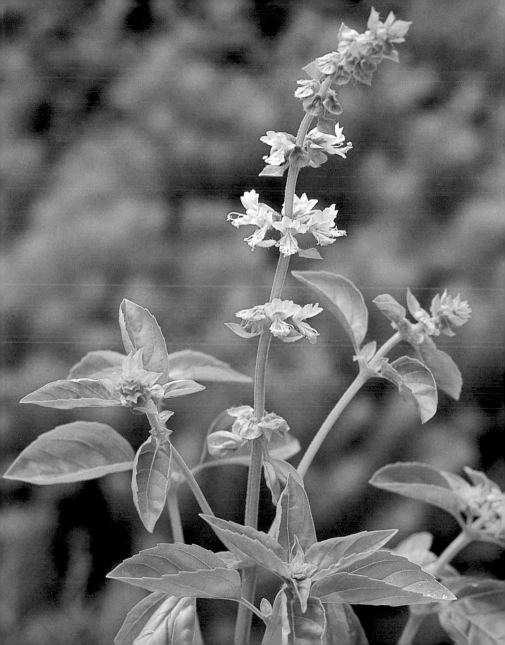

Green Jasper (ALASKA)

− INDICATIONS

uneven flow of sexual energy

trauma of sexual abuse

ungrounded, weak, or lost connection with the earth

stagnation or "constipation" of energy in the lower body

+ EFFECTS

opens you up to the "energy and grace of the wild feminine"

helps restore earthy sexuality

promotes a healthy sensuality

reestablishes and synchronizes the body's rhythms

Stagnated energy in the lower body means, in esoteric terms, that there is not much life force or vitality powering through the body's sexual and creative (sacral) center, so sexual enthusiasm and drive may be low or even nonexistent. Green Jasper (a gem essence) can restore a healthy flow of energy through the body's sexual center, and is also said to help women, especially older ones, to let go of their seriousness and replace it with a refreshing dose of sheer naughtiness.

Floral Caju (BRA)

− INDICATIONS

menopause and andropause

the ending of any sexual life-cycle

sadness

lack of energy

low in creativity

fertility problems

potency problems

+ EFFECTS

transforms a "stagnant" time into a rebirth

helps you find a new level or type of sensuality

promotes creativity and fertility

stimulates vitality and happiness

This essence helps you see and understand how each cycle of life can and does bring creative, new, and different ways to develop sensuality with pleasure and imagination. It is often used for men or women reaching midlife who feel their sexual rhythms and needs changing, and may be looking for additional outlets for their creative energy as well as still wishing to express themselves through their sexuality. Floral Caju is also given to women to support them during pregnancy.

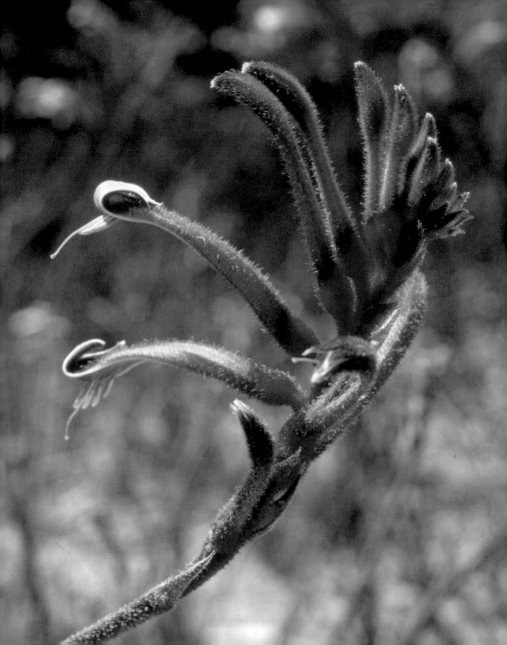

Love

Essences can be a wonderful support for every sort of love, including the romantic partner-to-partner variety. They also help heal the heart chakra, the energy center in the chest that is the seat of our emotions — remember how it feels when your heart literally aches with sorrow, or softens and soars when you see someone you adore? This chakra can become blocked or damaged by emotional hurt and may shut down to protect itself, making it difficult for you to either give or receive love anymore. These essences can help open a heart that is closed in this way, and soothe many of its wounds.

Red & Green Kangaroo Paw
(AUS)

— INDICATIONS
drifting away from your loved ones
loving partners who are becoming like roommates
working parents experiencing growing distance between
themselves and their children
you are unaware of how out of touch you are becoming

+ EFFECTS
helps you make time and space for closeness again
facilitates your coming back together

This essence is for couples who find that work is getting in the way of their relationship — especially if the harshness of the workaday world is becoming a part of them. It is also for those who cannot leave the world at the door when they come home. Both of you should take it if you are becoming estranged. If one or both of you just wants to be left alone when you return home, try Red Leschenaultia instead. If most or even all of the above sounds familiar, combine the two (see Living Essences' website/book on pages 297/302 for details, since, unlike other ranges, anything from 3 to 70 drops of this collection's essences are used).

Wild Horse (USA)

— INDICATIONS

brokenhearted

depressed, sad

lonely

children who have been emotionally hurt

if you feel you've lost heart with life, something, or someone

+ EFFECTS

supports the mending of a broken heart

produces a sense of being "heartened"

encourages the feeling of a loving belonging with others

helps you experience a connection with others

engenders loving emotional strength and power

Wild Horse is a true heart tonic, helping the heart chakra — the seat of all your emotions — to open gently so that you can love yourself and others, while at the same time nurturing your own healthy feelings of strength and power. It is very helpful for those who feel unhappy after breaking up with a partner, and is also good for supporting the healing of emotional damage of all kinds. (See also Butterfly page 239 and Bottlebrush page 244.)

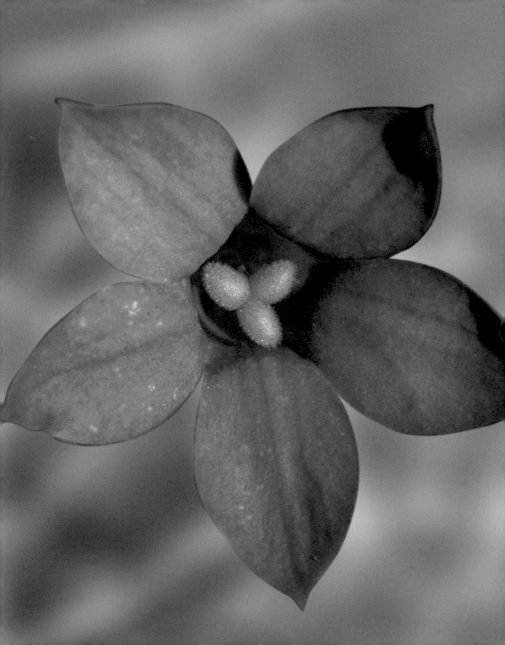

Bluebell (AUS)

— INDICATIONS

believing your supply of love may run out if you give too much away

fearing that love is a finite thing

living in fear of lack

your heart is closed off

you have a controlled, rigid, overly forthright manner

for young children who won't share their toys

after heart surgery

+ EFFECTS

encourages trust and joyful sharing

brings the knowledge that there is plenty to go around

opens up the heart to love

may support a swifter recovery from heart surgery

If you find loving difficult because some part of you fears that if you give your love away there will be nothing left and you won't survive, this essence is for you. It is also used following heart surgery, as it helps people to release old emotions that they have held onto for years — these tend to be kept around the heart area, thereby blocking it. Cardiac units note that postoperative heart patients who are able to cry freely (a good way of releasing emotional backlogs) tend to recover more quickly — and Bluebell can support this.

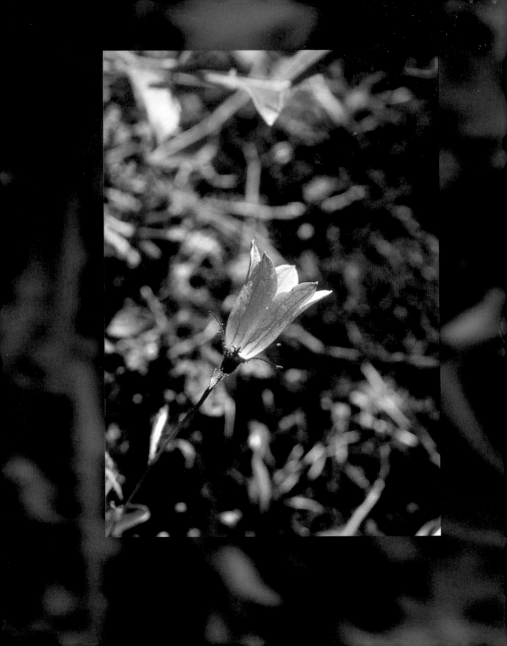

Harebell <small>(ALASKA)</small>

— INDICATIONS

desperately searching for love outside yourself
believing you can only get love from other people
fearing there's not enough love to go around
can't share your love, because you don't feel cherished by another
unable to receive the love that is available

+ EFFECTS

helps you let in Universal Love
shows you that this is limitless and inexhaustible
invites you to look inside yourself, too, for the love you need
encourages unconditional love to flow from you to others

Harebell essence helps you redefine your perceptions of love. It challenges the idea that "you can only get this from others, and so love must be both conditional and bound by many limitations and waiver," which can prevent you from ever being able to receive the kind or amount of love you need. It is interesting that in many essence ranges it is bluebells, and their relatives such as the harebells, which time and again are used to make remedies that will support you in many different aspects of loving and issues of the heart.

Penta (USA)

— INDICATIONS
you tend to withhold love
are fearful of needing others
believe that love hurts
may be seen as selfish or inconsiderate

+ EFFECTS
allows you to feel safe enough to give love to another
enables you to receive it back again
creates a healthy, independent way of loving

Penta personalities have learned through bitter past experience to rely
only on themselves, yet this essence can ease the pain that they carry with
them. Then, once they feel safe enough to love, they can be wonderful
partners — and terrific examples of how to be healthily independent in a
loving relationship by relying more on themselves for their needs, instead
of inadvertently draining those they love in order to nurture themselves.

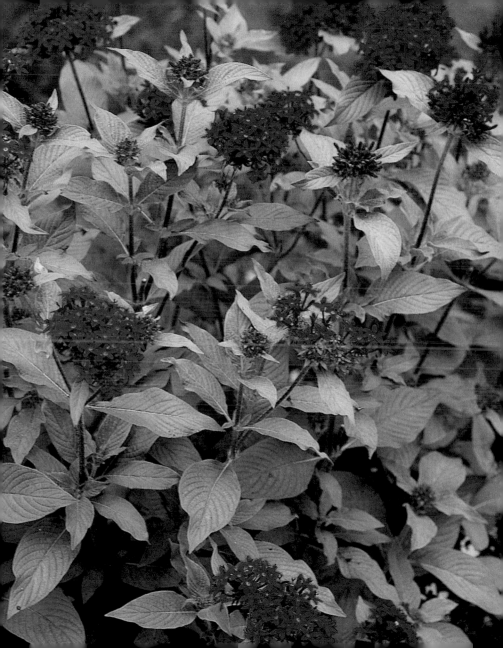

Love Essence (EIRE)

— INDICATIONS

a difficult child is causing emotional tension between the parents
love is becoming submerged beneath tiredness, frustration, and anger
stress caused by this child is affecting the entire family negatively
there is growing resentment of the child, who is labeled "the patient"

+ EFFECTS

encourages you to remember how much you love this child
renews your ability to show this, so that you can let love back in again
helps restore whole-family peace, balance, and harmony
improves the relationship between the parents

This combination gem essence is one for all the family to take together if there is one particular child who needs a lot of extra help, or is so disruptive that the entire family revolves around that child's needs and negative aspects. These problems may be due to the child's learning difficulties, mental illness, emotional problems, physical disability, or addiction. Without meaning to, such a high-need son or daughter can place an enormous strain on their parents' relationship, as well as on the dynamics of the family as a whole. However, this essence can help by exerting a powerful loving and softening effect on the way all family members relate to each other. Besides taking it orally, it's great to spray around the house to lift the atmosphere.

Pom Pom Tree (S AF)

— INDICATIONS
hiding feelings behind a front of self-sufficiency
"*I don't need anyone*"
refusing to allow anyone to get close
terror of letting yourself be vulnerable
extreme fear of rejection

+ EFFECTS
helps develop the courage that allows you to let others in
enables you to risk warm human contact
promotes the courage to allow closeness
brings emotional healing

This essence is for anyone who avoids closeness and intimacy with others, because they are afraid that if someone really gets to know them they may somehow be found wanting — and the loved one will then leave. It is also a remedy of choice if you are ashamed of certain aspects of yourself, and worry that if others discover these you will be rejected or abandoned: something that may have happened to you before. Pom Pom Tree can also be used for a deep, painful fear of rejection based upon intense childhood or past-life trauma.

Magnolia (UK)

— INDICATIONS

rigid ideas about love — it must be like this, or that
uncertainty about love at every level
believing that receiving love is conditional on good behavior

+ EFFECTS

awakens the power of unconditional love
brings the understanding that real love can hurt, but accepting this freely
clears away complications around situations involving love
simplifies the giving and receiving of love of all types

Magnolia is the essence that mirrors pure, unconditional love: the sort that has no boundaries, no strings, that conquers everything, and whose sheer power is limitless and awe-inspiring. This kind of true love is not necessarily easy, comfortable, and sweet. In fact, it can be disturbing to be on the receiving end, for it is very different from the sentimentality that often passes for love, and will at times be a double-edged sword which may be cutting for the greater good.

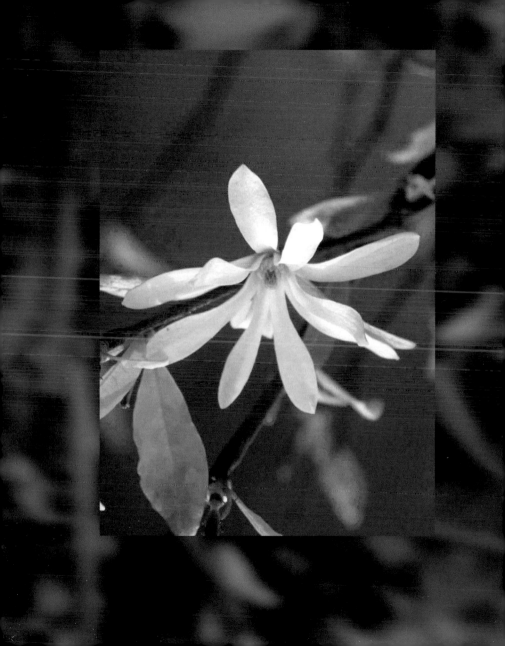

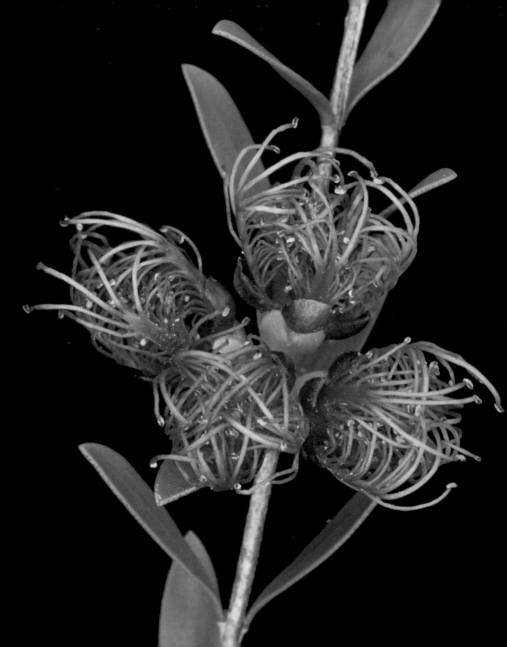

Mauve Melaleuca (Aus)

— INDICATIONS

you have given love, but not received it

you're a "hurt giver"

your own needs for love are not being met

you are trying to find love with the wrong people — who hurt you

your disappointment causes anger, sadness, frustration, even spite

+ EFFECTS

helps heal sadness and hurt

boosts self-assurance and self-containment

enables you to find new inner contentment

shows you that love lies within, and so is always with you

unconditional love

For those who have freely given their love, but feel very hurt because they have been offered none in return. They may have become angry, even spiteful, for they cannot see why the other person(s) won't respond. Also for children who lack parental love, lovers who receive none from their partners, loving parents whose children don't return their love. It helps them find the depths of the love for which they long inside themselves and to know that this can never leave them. This encourages unconditional love and freedom from expectations and dependency, as well as self-assurance and a happy disposition, allowing hurt feelings to heal.

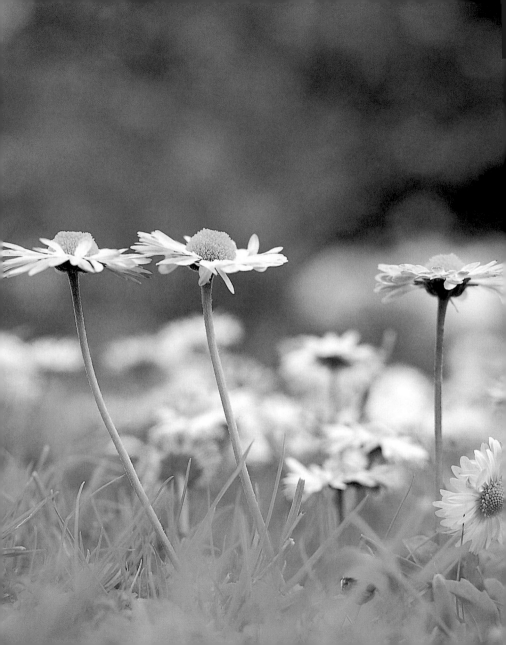

Children

Bursting with limitless potential, love, curiosity, and wisdom, children are far, far more than the embryonic adults we often treat them as being. It is our task as adults to protect, love, and support our children as they become acquainted with this planet and how it works. Openhearted, psychically aware, adaptable yet vulnerable, children develop fast at all levels from birth to age 18 while remaining at the mercy of the adult world. They may need very particular kinds of support at different times to help them cope with the challenges they'll meet on their journey. In this way, they will develop into happy, confident young adults who are able to use their remarkable individual gifts to achieve the potential with which they were born.

Daisy

Daisy (UK)

— INDICATIONS

off-balance, giddy, bewildered

distracted, scatterbrained, flighty

out of control

overwhelmed

capricious, fickle, easily swayed

nervous, oversensitive

+ EFFECTS

enables the child to respond to situations, rather than just reacting

insures they are grounded and centered

helps them feel protected and safe

encourages playfulness

Daisy supports children (and adults) by grounding them when they've been overwhelmed by a situation or event. It helps them detach themselves from any outer turmoil — for this essence is soothing, quietening, and calming to the nerves. Daisy is an excellent remedy when events may have made you feel as if the rug has been pulled out from under your feet, or when former certainties and securities have suddenly been taken away. Taking it after a fraught or busy day can also be a great help. (A very good way for a child to take it is to have a warm bath with some drops of Daisy in it.)

The Works <small>(EIRE)</small>

— INDICATIONS

in crisis

existential distress: "What am I doing here?"

for children or teenagers verging on the suicidal

something is all wrong, but the child doesn't know what

being bullied

+ EFFECTS

offers emotional rescue

enables the child to identify what's wrong, so they can begin to address it

helps them remember the point of it all

stabilizes

calms

The Works can be especially helpful to teenagers who are in turmoil or who have reached breaking point. When they are literally locked in their rooms and cannot or will not come out to take part in the world, this combination gem essence can help draw them out so that you can work with them on the cause of their distress. This process may involve not only supporting and talking to them at home, but also finding a professional therapist whom the child likes and is willing to talk to.

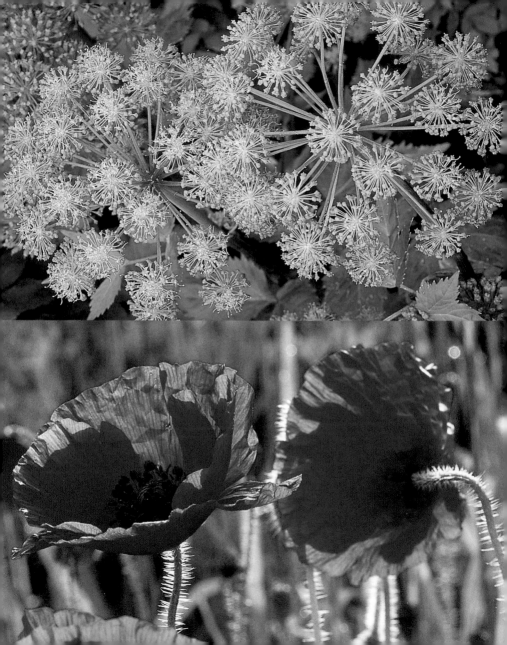

Love (NLD)

— INDICATIONS

self-confidence at rock bottom

feeling suicidal

cannot receive love from parents

going through puberty

for all heart problems — emotional and physical

+ EFFECTS

enhances the child's sense of self-worth

helps them to love themselves

allows them to do things for others from sheer love

shows the child how to enjoy and love life

encourages them to love their physical body

This is one of the most profound and loving essence combinations for adults as well as children, for it connects us all with our own inner self and source — with who we truly are. As with many essences supporting issues of the heart, Love is also said to be helpful for anyone undergoing heart surgery, as it encourages more rapid healing and may reduce postoperative shock.

Wattle (AUS)

— INDICATIONS

for teenagers who:
don't see how vulnerable they make themselves to harm
display shallow naïveté
aren't thinking about the consequences of their behavior
make fun of caution, rebel against taking care
leap into situations for which they're not ready
act scattily
show indifference to important information

+ EFFECTS

fosters alertness and mental awareness
encourages a mature and wise view of life
brings understanding about avoiding unnecessary dangers
provides a steadying influence

This essence clarifies the wisdom of good choices and the consequences of bad ones so that you can explore life, have fun, and experience adventure — without danger. Wattle helps teenagers face up to the realities of life, one of which is that naïveté doesn't protect anyone from the consequences of their own decisions. The beginning of the short meditation that goes with Wattle is: *"Today I know but little, tomorrow I will know more. Each step will bring me closer to understanding."*

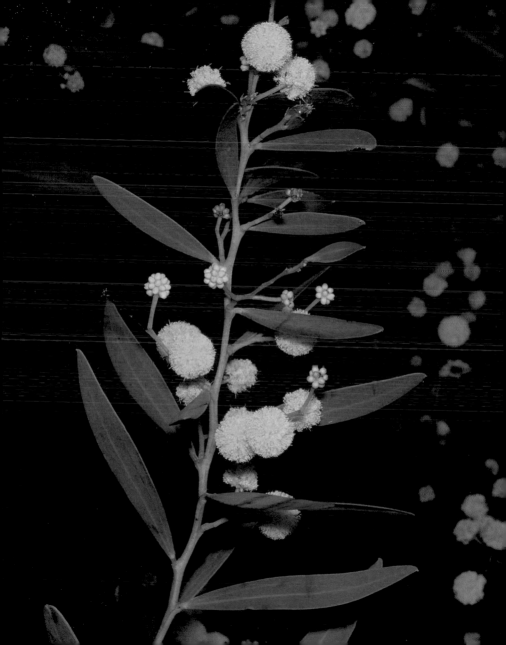

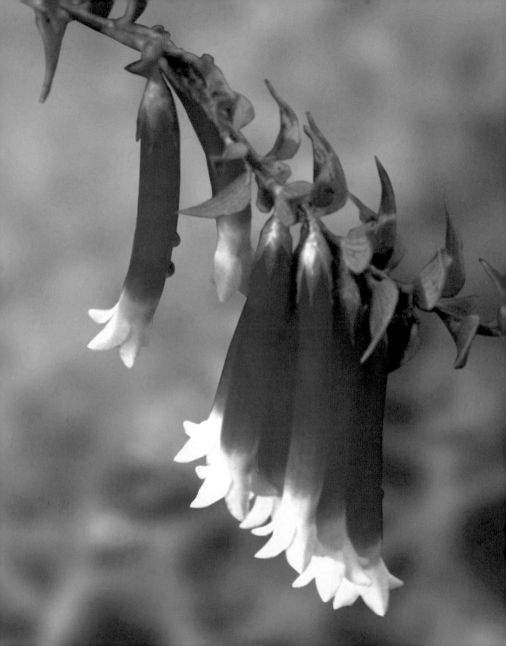

Bush Fuchsia (AUS)

— INDICATIONS

dyslexia, dyspraxia, Attention Deficit Disorder with Hyperactivity

difficulty decoding others' social cues

poor learning ability

stuttering, speech hesitancy

cannot read for long before losing concentration

inability to trust own intuition

+ EFFECTS

promotes clarity and confidence in speaking

fosters a better balance between left and right sides of the brain

improves concentration

helps the child read more easily and write more clearly

encourages better awareness and processing of others' social signals

For learning disorders where left/right side of brain is impaired. For dyslexia and dyspraxia, the suggested regime is to take Bush Fuchsia for two to four weeks, break for two weeks, then take it for another two weeks. The remedy can be used like this for weeks or months, gradually phasing it out. It is helpful, too, when the child feels dull or switched off after spending a lot of time in front of video games or other electronic equipment. For general learning enhancement, try Cognis (which contains Bush Fuchsia); to improve social skills, try Kangaroo Paw.

Hiddenite and Kunzite *(Eire)*

— INDICATIONS
difficulty connecting with others emotionally
unsure how to behave with them
not sure how to be on the planet at all
feeling like a space cadet, apart, different
filled with sadness

+ EFFECTS
promotes easier relationships
helps the child communicate and connect with others
if things have been hard, shows the child they can be happy again
enables them to make friends more easily

This is the "feeling part of things" essence — for those who often feel like an alien on their own planet. It is no coincidence that one of the stones this remedy is made from is a damaged little gem that looks like a spaceship but whose colors are those of the heart — pink and green. It helps show space cadets, who do not find it easy to connect with others but would like a close friend (or partner), how to "plug in." This essence is also helpful for children with Asperger's syndrome, and for teenagers (especially boys) embarking on first relationships.

Calling all Angels *(ALASKA)*

— INDICATIONS

not feeling safe, especially at night

not feeling "at home" in your own bedroom

unsettled, nervous

difficulty falling asleep

broken sleep

bad dreams and nightmares

+ EFFECTS

offers peace and protection

encourages deep, restful sleep

provides a feeling of softness and serenity

accesses the protection, love, and guidance of angels

produces a safe, calm atmosphere in your own room

This wonderful combination of Angelica, Chalice Well, Chiming Bells, and Kunzite creates a soft, serene atmosphere: lovely for misting around a child's room before bedtime, taking internally, or adding (two drops) to the evening bath. Chiming Bells helps connect everyone with the real, tangible source of spiritual support that is always available, no matter how lost they may be feeling. Chalice Well is made from the sacred well in Glastonbury, England, and again it connects us to the powerful spiritual and angelic support beyond our current awareness.

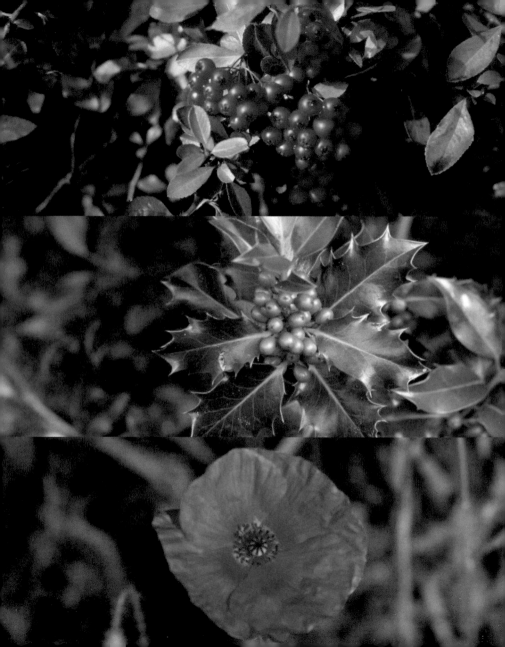

Anger and Frustration

(UK)

— INDICATIONS

flies into a rage easily

finds it difficult to control anger when in the midst of it

low flashpoint

goes into "self-destruct" mode out of sheer frustration

turns anger inward

+ EFFECTS

balances

helps prevent the child from rising to the bait so easily

takes the sting out of situations

offers the child more control over their fire energy

helps them to grasp situations more accurately and respond better

Fire energy is the driving force behind everything we do. Too little of it and we become ineffective, too much and we become destructive. Fire that has got out of hand can be harmful to both ourselves and others, so it needs to be stabilized and kept under our own control. This combination essence — a mixture of Red Poppy, Firethorn, and Holly Leaf — is helpful for toddler tantrums, for adolescents who have trouble handling any rage and resentment, and for children of any age who experience difficulties controlling their response to feeling angry.

Maple *(S AF)*

— INDICATIONS

periods of major physical growth, such as the teenage years
difficulty managing and/or coordinating the growing body
burning the candle at both ends
using willpower to keep going — to the point of physical depletion

+ EFFECTS

achieves a balance between physical growth and
the developing personality
offers a gentle containment without stricture or confinement
supports children whose bodies temporarily outstrip their coordination

This essence is particularly helpful for adolescents, especially if they are going through a period of rapid emotional or physical development (the gangly, all-arms-and-legs period) or when they have a surge in body mass and strength but do not yet seem in control of or even comfortable with it. Maple is also useful for workaholics or the overly goal-oriented and it can support teenagers who are being pushed to do too much, perhaps in school at times leading up to important examinations.

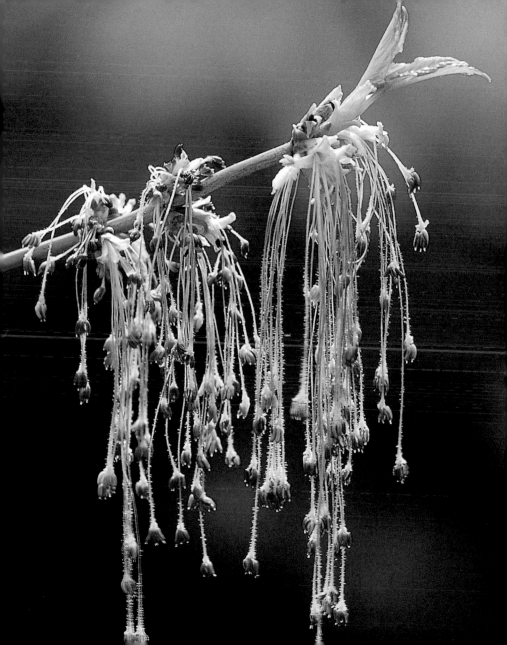

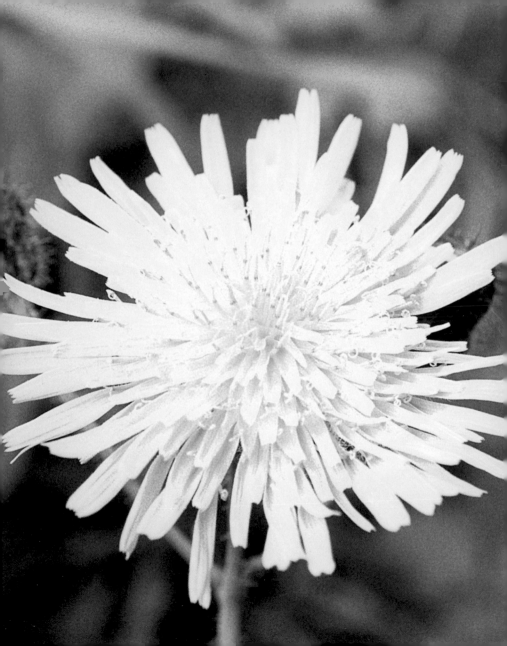

Father Sun (UK)

— INDICATIONS

children in single-parent families whose father is absent
teenagers/early 20's lacking confidence about managing in the world
male teens/early 20's with little sense of direction
boys growing up without a strong, caring male role model
children or adults who have/had fathers who do/did not cope well with life
children grieving from loss or anticipated loss of a father or father figure

+ EFFECTS

helps the child move out into the world and deal with it with assurance
helps them see who they are and what they can do
encourages a strong, positive male identity for boys/very young men
supports them to leave home with confidence and manage well
enables them to comfort, support, and counsel themselves

Made from the common hawkweed, this essence is helpful for young people who feel vulnerable, lacking in strength, or fearful of not being able to cope on their own in the world. Both boys and girls need an inspiring, caring male role model, especially from age seven to adulthood, to motivate, praise, and support their development. Father Sun helps them to embody the lionhearted masculine radiance of the Sun, so that they feel robust and confident enough to deal with life out there.

Mercutio (UK)

— INDICATIONS

for children or teenagers who are being bullied
too embroiled in events to see what's going on, and how best to react
are not very articulate; verbally adept kids run rings around them
feel frustrated
lack social ease
take things too seriously

+ EFFECTS

brings poise and humor
enhances word-play ability and verbal repartee skills
encourages children not to take life, or themselves, so seriously
improves the understanding of interplay between people, and of dialogue
invites sheer enjoyment of the movement of words, and their meaning

This essence was named after Mercutio, a character in Shakespeare's *Romeo and Juliet*, a great word-play artist and sophisticated social animal who possessed polish, humor, courage, and ease by the bucketload. It helps children to stand back a bit from the drama of life whether in the playground or at home, and achieve a calmer overview of what's going on, the better to be able to consider their reactions and respond appropriately. It is also said to bring positive energy ("white light") to the eyes, so may be helpful if a child or teenager is reading or studying a lot.

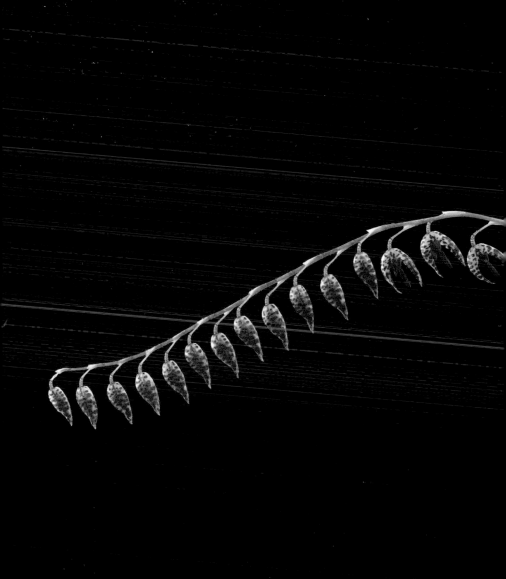

Balancer <small>(CAN)</small>

— INDICATIONS

the child has forgotten the source of their distress, but just feels miserable

they are agitated

all over the place

overtired, exhausted

disorientated

+ EFFECTS

balances

calms

encourages the child to take the rest they need

restores perspective

Balancer is described as being "like immersing yourself in a soothing, cooling waterfall and emerging rejuvenated and refreshed," and it can be used for coping with many different stressful situations. Also try Dolphin for any child separated from those they love for whatever reason, such as hospitalization, being orphaned, having to live apart from their own family (for example, for temporarily fostered children). For children struggling with the impact of separating or divorced parents, or other challenges to their sense of safety, another essence, called Heart Spirit, can be both helpful and supportive.

Just Me (UK)

— INDICATIONS

for children who feel different from their peers
don't feel good enough, or not as good as their friends
don't feel special in a positive way, or feel undervalued
have not been loved, or don't feel themselves to be loved
feel as if they don't fit in
are not comfortable with themselves

+ EFFECTS

helps a child accept themselves: "This is who I am"
brings the knowledge that they are just fine the way they are
supports those who don't fit into the neat slots society provides for them
celebrates their own uniqueness
brings acceptance that limitations are life stages, not something negative

This essence can support the growing number of children who just don't fit the existing mold, question everything, see too much, have a different slant on life — and may therefore be labeled difficult, geeky, or weird. Some may be Indigo Children, a new type of wise child that is coming through who will help the planet move forward as it must, but who find life and its conventional restrictions difficult. Initially a puzzle to many parents, these children can become an inspiration and delight to all who are part of their lives.

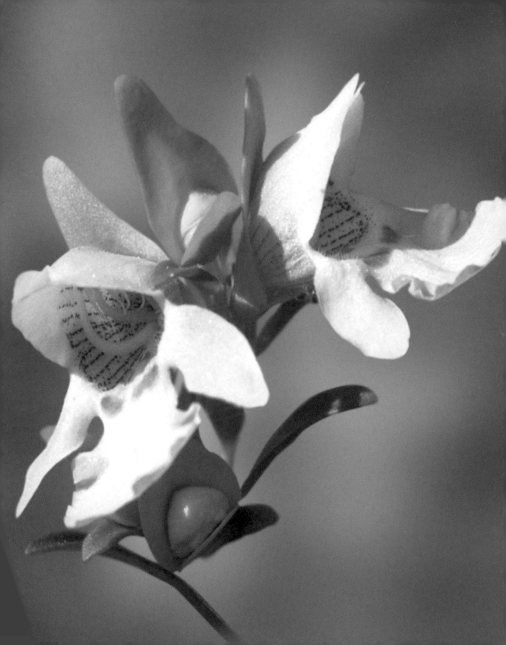

Nurturers

Those who dedicate their lives to looking after others may find they feel a very particular sort of tiredness, one that goes way beyond what even office workers clocking up punishing hours may experience. Burnout is the major depletion of your physical, emotional, and perhaps also spiritual resources, caused by giving of yourself 24/7. Parents of young children, caregivers of live-in elderly relatives, and those in the front line of professions such as doctors, nurses, social workers, and therapists are especially vulnerable to this. The following essences can help you to recover, but will also support you in looking at your situation so you can see how you got there, and assess what you could do to insure you never become this exhausted again.

ALPINE MINT BUSH

Alpine Mint Bush (AUS)

— INDICATIONS

carer fatigue

parental burnout

practitioner fatigue

mental and emotional weariness

feeling weighed down by responsibility

the "Why bother?" feeling

+ EFFECTS

renews, revitalizes

brings in joy

enables you to consider how to balance your life

For caregivers of all types who feel more than physical exhaustion —
including parents of very young or disabled children, and those looking
after ill partners or older parents. This essence can help you assess the
way you are using your energies. It is also appropriate for professional
burnout among doctors or therapists (encouraging a reevaluation of
working practices) and others in careers where they have to make
constant choices about the welfare of others but in a more detached role
than that of such caregivers as social workers. Alpine Mint Bush can also
help you to establish healthy boundaries, and say "No" more often. Try to
use it preventively *before* you begin to feel burned out.

Robin (USA)

— INDICATIONS

expending a lot of energy nurturing others
forgetting that you need to be looked after, too
discord and stress at home
for parents who would like to be better caregivers
supports children who have been hurt by their parents
for those who have unresolved issues with their mothers

+ EFFECTS

encourages you to nurture and love yourself
supports your ability to be a loving parent
enhances family harmony
helps you create peace and accord out of chaos

Robin is the family and nurturing essence. It can help new parents who may feel overwhelmed or intimidated by their task, encourage new mothers and fathers to connect and bond with their babies, and support mothers after a difficult or traumatic birth. It is also a good general remedy for parents during difficult times with their children. But perhaps one of the most important ways in which Robin can be used is as a powerful aid for helping you learn to nurture and parent yourself.

Sycamore (UK)

— INDICATIONS

stressed, stretched to breaking point
worn down over time
profound fatigue and exhaustion
spiritually testing times

+ EFFECTS

taps into your inner reserves of strength
acts as a catalyst for renewed energy
encourages continuity of effort
promotes flexibility and resilience under stress
helps you set boundaries
supports you in saying "No" when you need to

Sycamore is an essence for when you are worn down by time, effort, or stress. It is helpful for those struggling to stay on top of family problems, for exhausted parents of children who are proving difficult to raise, and for caregivers of elderly parents. It is also a good remedy for the exhaustion caused by less emotionally charged personal issues, such as difficult or uncertain times at work or convalescence after a long illness.

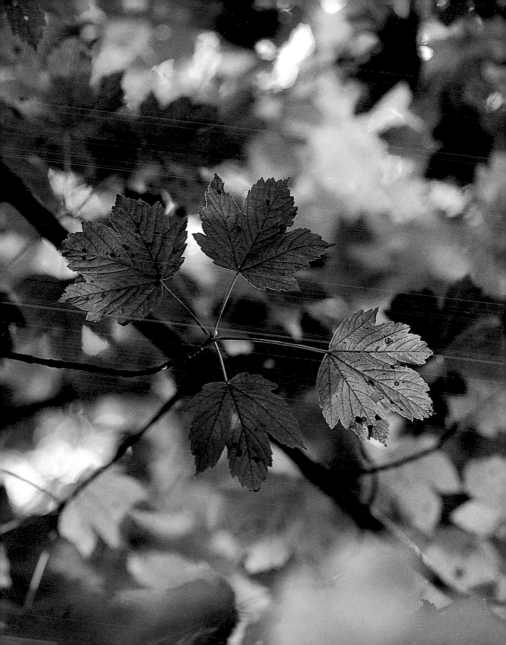

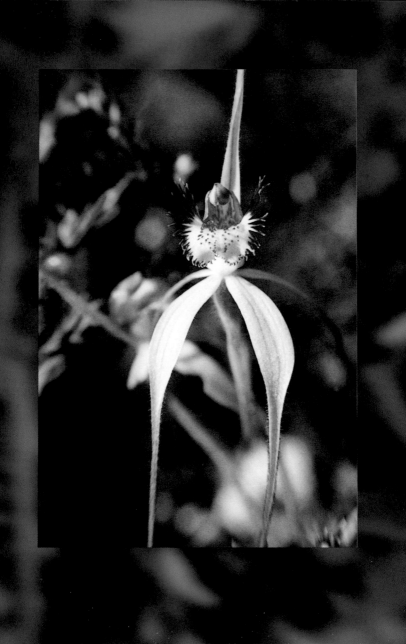

White Spider Orchid (AUS)

— INDICATIONS

for humanitarian workers struggling to cope with the distress they see
oversensitivity to the pain of others
for caregivers who cannot go on
for people whose high ideals have been abused
you are aware of others' pain, but feel paralyzed by it

+ EFFECTS

facilitates empathy with the distress of others, without being derailed by it
promotes the ability to relieve suffering without burning out yourself

This essence is for the overwhelmed humanitarian, and it supports those seeking to make this world a better place. It helps inspire people in the front line of the caring and volunteer services, whether in a war-torn third-world country or a local refuge home. White Spider Orchid can bring the suffering many volunteers see every day into perspective by offering an overview of the reason for pain in a soul's individual journey, thereby making it less traumatic to witness and easier to help.

Cyclamen (UK)

— INDICATIONS

allowing your life to be governed by external demands

loss of sense of self

anger and resentment

putting your own life and happiness on hold

feeling as if all your creativity/inspiration has evaporated

lack of fulfillment

exhaustion, burnout

+ EFFECTS

enables you to create time for yourself

helps you create a rich and satisfying life

encourages you to look after yourself properly (which also
benefits those around you)

Cyclamen is about having a life *now*, rather than at some point in the
future, by which time you may be too exhausted by life-stress to enjoy it.
This essence helps you be kind to yourself. It can also support you in
taking a good look at the life you are creating, so that you can think about
whether this is what you really want — and if it isn't, Cyclamen can help
you work out what you might need instead.

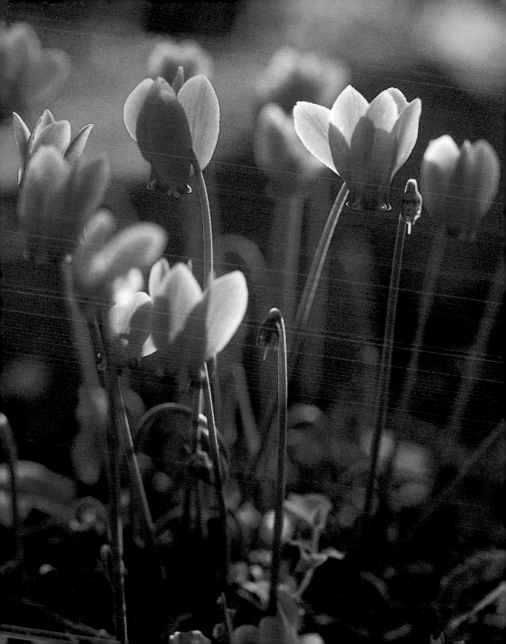

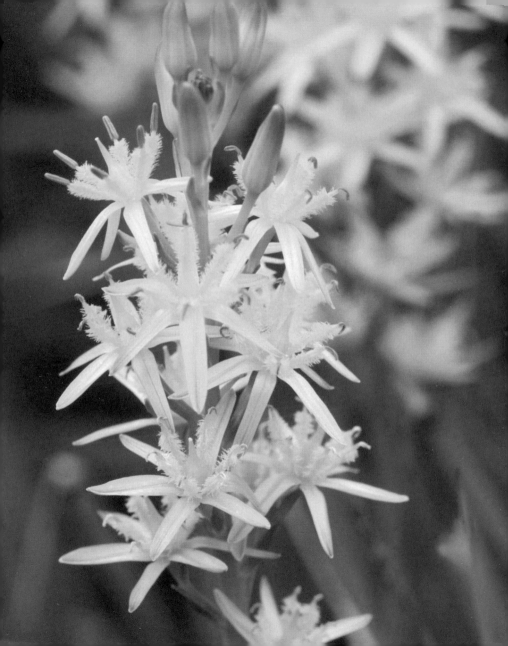

Bog Asphodel (UK)

— INDICATIONS

an overpowering ambition to help other people
cannot see that those you help may need to work out
their salvation for themselves
feel trapped by your own reaction to the distress of others
for the willing servant, or slave

+ EFFECTS

helps you take your mission in life more lightly
encourages you to avoid entanglements in the suffering of others
releases you from feeling trapped by your work
enhances your ability to consider your own situation
enables you to look at your own personal development and growth

This essence helps you understand that if you impose your help on others, you may actually be doing them a disservice by blocking their own healing process. The truth is that real help for others comes from a natural overflowing of their own strengths and wisdom. And while they may welcome a degree of support from you when it is necessary, your own enthusiasm and strong opinions about what you believe they need are no substitute for this realization of their own inner resources.

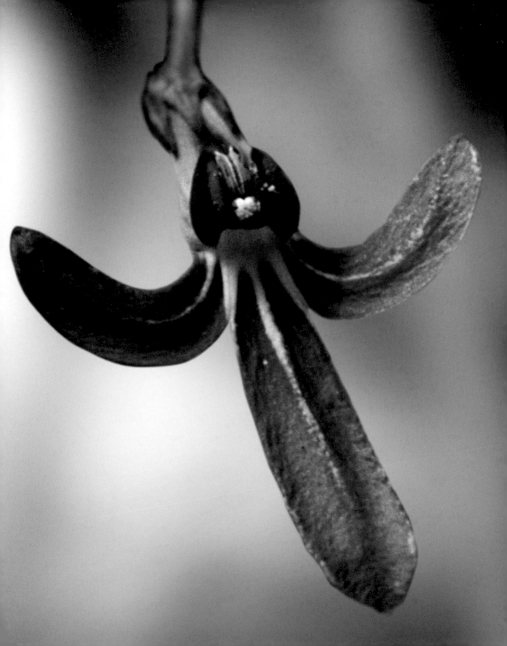

Purification

Purification may initially sound a little saintly, but in fact is thoroughly down-to-earth and practical — the basis for feeling good physically, and for being "clear" for self-development and/or further spiritual progression.

Purification may be needed on several levels: physically (perhaps you live in a polluted area), emotionally (possibly following abuse, which has left you feeling soiled and dirtied), or spiritually (perhaps a deep past-life issue, or maybe having been with someone very negative or unpleasant). If you cannot see any single essence here that rings a bell but you feel you need a "clearout," consider a good general combination such as Aura Cleaning, Purification Formula, or Purity.

Angelsword (Aus)

— INDICATIONS

contamination with negative energy, often other people's
spiritual possession
gullibility about spiritual issues and information received

+ EFFECTS

cleanses very powerfully
insures that any spiritual guidance you receive is
clear, accurate, and truthful

If you've had a bad day or been in contact with people who have left
you feeling negative or contaminated (which may manifest as feeling
unusually drained, irritable, anxious, and out of sorts), a very effective
way to use Angelsword is to supplement or substitute oral treatment
by putting six to ten drops in a bath and soaking for at least ten minutes,
feeling all the negativity of the day dissolve. Consider also Wild Potato
Bush if you are detoxing your body of heavy metals such as lead, or
mercury from old amalgam fillings, and Billy Goat Plum (see page 139),
if you are feeling defiled sexually.

Obaiti (BRA)

— INDICATIONS

a sense of impurity
feeling "contaminated," emotionally toxic
difficulty eliminating physical wastes or toxins

+ EFFECTS

helps remove the emotional and spiritual debris that
accumulates over a lifetime
cleanses and releases old patterns
liberates you from old or redundant ways of behaving

This essence is made from the aerial roots of a plant that grows on the Atlantic coast of Brazil, and contains water from the ocean rather than from a land source. The affirmation that goes with it is, *"I free myself from old patterns that block my growth"*, and its key word is "liberation." Obaiti is also used to help bring focus to any issue you have been mulling over, perhaps for some time. In addition, it is often prescribed if you are having trouble studying, perhaps when examinations are looming or when your academic workload has become both heavier and more demanding.

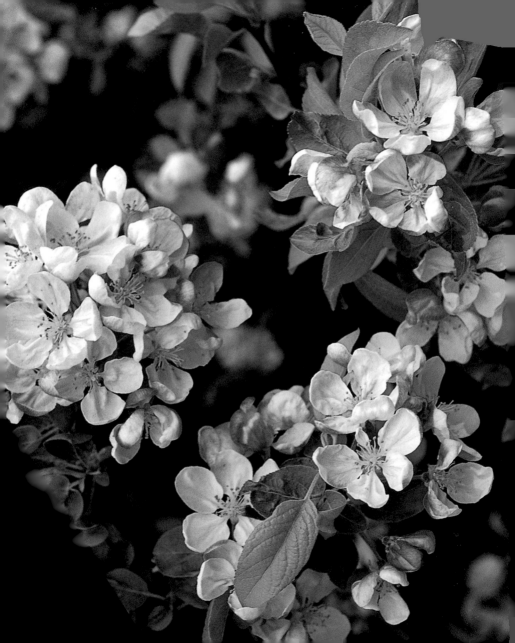

Crab Apple *(UK)*

— INDICATIONS

feel dirtied, besmirched, grubby

great need for cleanliness, such as repeated washing of self

great need for order: perhaps obsessively tidy at home

very distressed by skin eruptions like pimples or rashes

afraid that foods may be "off," public restrooms filthy, germs everywhere

possible problems with activities such as breastfeeding or deep kissing

+ EFFECTS

cleanses on both a mental and a physical level

helps you accept your imperfections

promotes a positive self-image

fosters a more relaxed attitude

restores your perspective

Sometimes used alongside fasting, Crab Apple is also suitable for hangovers (four drops every 30 minutes) and to help calm skin problems such as pimples or heat rash, where it may be used both orally and topically. Some practitioners suggest this essence to help combat the side effects of certain drugs, such as antibiotics. It is often taken to help remove negative impressions — for instance, after a dirty job or difficult personal-care nursing task. You can also use Crab Apple with Rescue Remedy to help treat pest-infested plants.

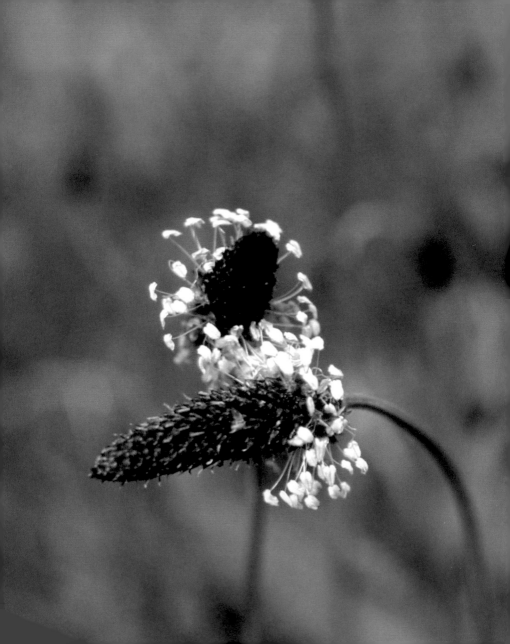

Plantain (CAN)

— INDICATIONS

thoughts and attitudes that feel as if they are poisoning you
frustration and resentment
repetitive thoughts over which you seem to have no control
bitterness and other negative emotional patterns
physical tension and rigidity

+ EFFECTS

brings emotional and spiritual cleansing
facilitates purification at all levels
enables you to let go of long-held physical tension

There are several different varieties of plantains — bananas, for example, whose fruits have long been used as a remedy for toxic snakebite, while herbalists traditionally use another type of plantain to make poultices for drawing out other poisons through the skin. Plantain essence works on the emotions and spirit in a similar way, but the venoms it draws out and releases are bitterness and resentment. As cleansing takes place on an emotional and spiritual level, therapists report that the body relaxes and loses its rigidity, too; for example, a long-standing pair of tight shoulders or jaws may soften and unclench.

Bladder Senna (UK)

− INDICATIONS

feeling clogged up with old energies

needing to escape from old patterns

carrying around baggage you no longer need

+ EFFECTS

brings a new "cleaned-out" feeling

helps expel old, outmoded energies

boosts your ability to jettison outdated burdens

This essence is the equivalent of a gentle but effective purgative at a physical level — and, indeed, senna taken in infusion or capsule form as a herbal remedy is an effective traditional treatment for physical constipation, or for a toxic gut that has become overloaded with old waste material. In the same way, the vibrational energy of Bladder Senna can help you get rid of accumulated waste at spiritual and emotional levels.

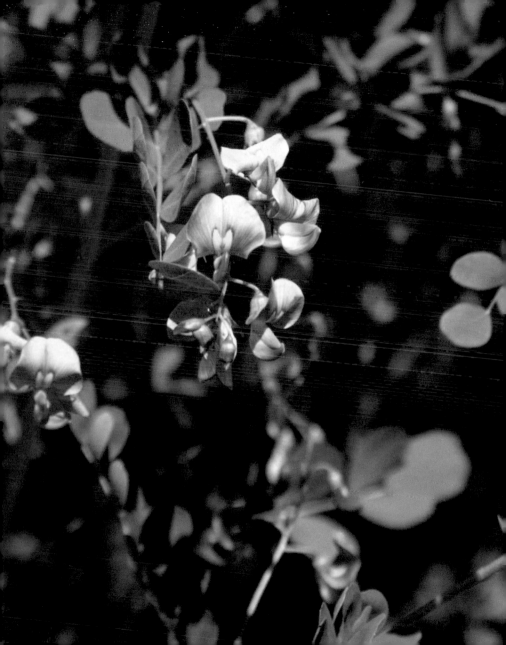

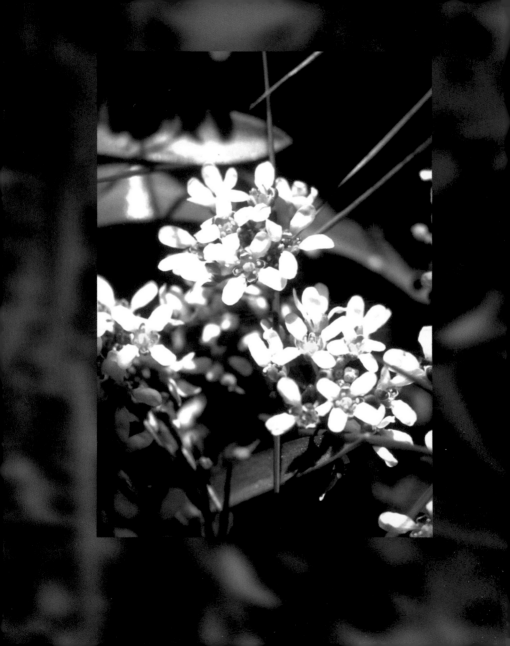

Watercress (UK)

— INDICATIONS

ill-health due to an unwholesome lifestyle or environment
neglecting your own wellbeing
contamination, toxicity
susceptibility to disease, low immunity, debilitation, miasmas
exposure to harmful substances or things

+ EFFECTS

purifies both the self and the environment
promotes clarification, purging, elimination, miasmatic clearing
facilitates drainage and discharge of dross and waste
works as an antiseptic, anti-inflammatory agent
helps strengthen the immune system and disease resistance
cools, soothes, calms

Watercress can have an anti-inflammatory effect at many different levels. It is good for "hot, festering wounds" and is often used for those who feel they are festering emotionally. It is also prescribed for sluggishness or stagnation of the life force or lifeblood, and purification of both the self and the environment — the underlying cause of which may be a weakness for substances or situations that are unwholesome but irresistible. In addition, it can help clear miasma (predispositions to recurrent, persistent, chronic, or inherited disease patterns).

Periwinkle (USA)

– INDICATIONS

feeling tied to a past experience
feeling held back by past events that happened in this
life you are leading now

+ EFFECTS

clears away experiences that are holding you back
helps cleanse and clear past life problems
clarifies your goals

Those who believe in past lives and reincarnation (and this covers most major world religions, including Christianity to the 5th century A.D.) feel there are often negative events or emotions held in people's "spiritual DNA" which may continue to affect you in your present life. This can prevent you from fulfilling your potential and trap you in past patterns of belief or behavior. Periwinkle can help wash away memories of those past experiences and beliefs, which dam the flow of your energy and hold you back from reaching your goals this time around. You may find your physical energy is renewed too, as blocked chi (life force) is released.

Portage Glacier (ALASKA)

— INDICATIONS

for places where there has been depression, addiction, conflict, or abuse
the atmosphere feels tired, stagnant, heavy
for toxic energies in the mind, emotions, and body
for places where people tend to argue, or lose vitality or focus easily
you are weighed down by (possibly others') depressing thoughts
a difficult period of physical detox

+ EFFECTS

acts as an excellent space clearer
helps release toxic energies from the mind, emotions, and physical body
purifies the feel of environments
is joyous, uplifting, liberating
recharges low energies

"Like a fountain of white light," this essence breaks up stagnant energy patterns: the first step in any space-clearing process. It is great for cleansing and revitalizing offices, meeting rooms, therapy rooms, refuge centers, hospitals, classrooms, healing spaces — and also for therapists themselves. Purification — the formula used by some hospitals as an addition to the cleaners' mop buckets when they wash the floors — also contains Portage Glacier. Consider also Grass of Parnassus, or Black Tourmaline gem essence, also ingredients of Purification.

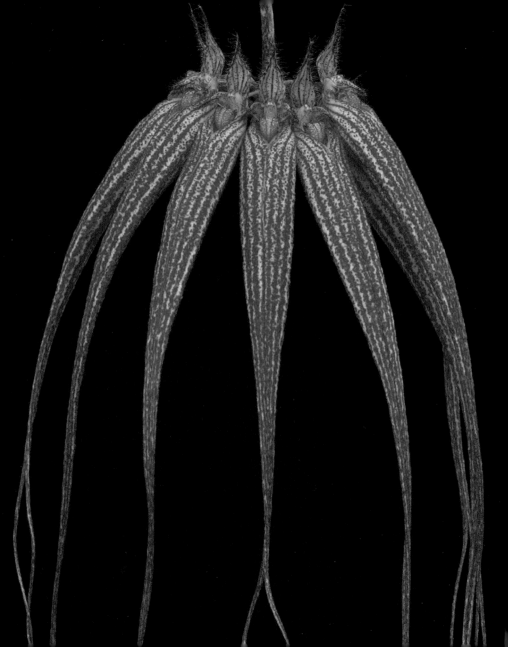

Protection

In a changing, challenging world, one of the
most important things you can do to feel safe,
no matter what is happening, is to insure that
you are protected and grounded. Grounding is
making your own energy connection with the
Earth: some visualize it literally as sending deep
"roots" down from their feet. Protection involves
creating a mental force field around yourself as
a barrier to negative energy. Some people use
the remarkable power of visualization, some
use geophysical methods such as magnets or
crystals, while others use affirmations or prayer.
Essences can be very effective either as adjuncts
to these measures, or used alone. Good
combinations include Yarrow Environmental
Solution, Psychic Protection, and Soul Shield.

Knight's Cloak (UK)

— INDICATIONS

attracting unwanted attention from negative people
for lightworkers/healers whose radiance is noticed by undesirable energies
being around those who want your energy
feeling vulnerable, unsafe
feeling exposed, overly visible

+ EFFECTS

helps you remain concealed from those who may threaten
promotes a sense of invisibility and invincibility
enables you to evade the attention of negative energies

Everyone radiates spiritual light, and the more "positive," spiritually developed, and clear someone is, the more light they will give out. You cannot usually see this with the naked eye, but you can sense it — perhaps as a good feeling around a person — and psychics may notice it as a visibly brighter aura. However, in darker times or periods of turbulence (like this) in humankind's development and our planet's evolution, it may well be wise to cloak your light to minimize the risk of attracting unwelcome attention from negative sources. Consider also the powerful Soul Shield combination, containing Knight's Cloak plus two other orchid essences: Pushing Back the Night and Protective Presence.

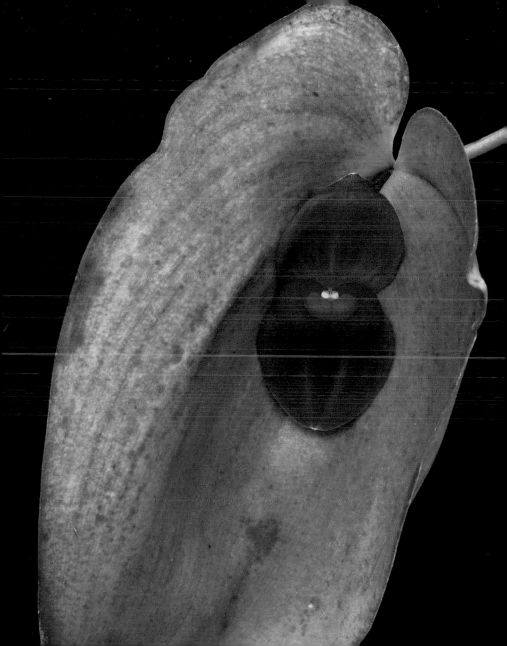

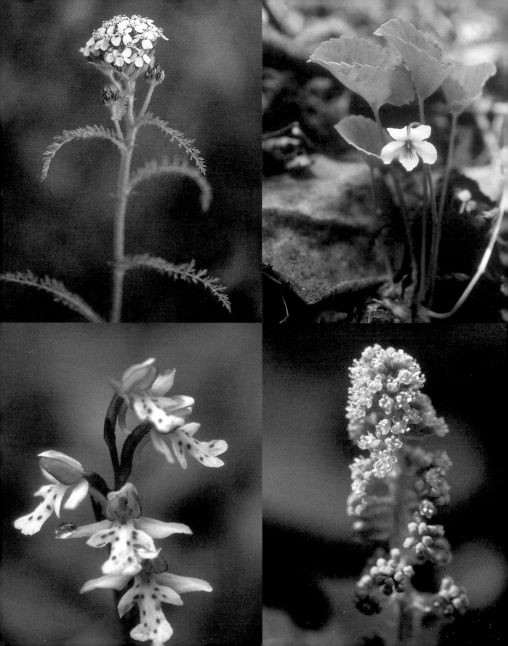

Guardian (ALASKA)

— INDICATIONS

working in a draining environment, such as a stressed office
finding yourself drained after contact with certain people
working around computers and other electronic equipment
feeling tired and run down
difficulty grounding in a new neighbouhood
you're doing healing work or space clearing/feng shui
for sensitive children who need protection while they build up their own

+ EFFECTS

allows you to feel safe
helps create a protective force field around you
encourages you to ground yourself strongly
empowers you to claim your space and create strong, healthy boundaries

Guardian is a terrific combination for anyone who is especially sensitive
to their surroundings or to the people around them, but who wishes to
become their own source of protection. It is invaluable for therapists and
counselors, for those working in stressful or competitive environments,
or people in front line jobs such as benefit offices, hospitals, refuge
centers, busy retail outlets, schools, airports, and the emergency services.
You can use Guardian both as a space-clearing and protection spray, and
as an essence to take internally or add to a warm bath.

Star Ruby (ALASKA)

— INDICATIONS

always straying off into your own thoughts
easily distracted
fantasizing or daydreaming a lot
resistant to being present in your body, especially
in challenging circumstances

+ EFFECTS

focuses you on the present moment
links you into what's happening *now*
helps you ground your awareness
penetrates resistance to being grounded — in your body or on the planet
energizes your roots, strengthening your connection with the earth

Star Ruby helps draw, attract, and anchor energy and information into the physical body. Several grounding essences are made, like this one, from the energy of gems, since the help offered to us by the mineral kingdom is structure and stability. Today, those who are becoming more interested in spiritual matters, or who are developing spiritually themselves, are also becoming more sensitive. Good grounding therefore becomes increasingly important, so that a growing ability to reach "upward," toward the Source of Light/God/the Divine can be matched by corresponding anchorage "downward."

Divine Being (UK)

— INDICATIONS

continuous fear of outside attack
constant anxiety about "harmful" external influences
feeling vulnerable, powerless
lack of belief in your own ability to heal and protect yourself

+ EFFECTS

brings the understanding that you are not just a weak mortal but
a powerful being of light energy
reinforces the knowledge that you can create your own reality with
your thoughts and beliefs
shows you that you can heal and defend yourself fully
helps you realize that you can be your own best protection
creates confidence in your own ability to heal

The spiritual Law of Attraction is that you draw to yourself that which you give out. This effectively means that if you expect attack, you will tend to attract it — but fortunately, it also means that the reverse is true, because you help create your own reality. This combination essence (*Achillea millefolium* and clear quartz) brings with it the knowledge that you are a being of spirit and nothing can harm your essential self. It also helps show you that your best protection comes from being at peace within yourself, and radiating that peace outward all around you.

Sundew (AUS)

— INDICATIONS

disconnected, "not really there"
vague, daydreaming life away
lacking in focus and attention to detail, procrastinating
fainting, coma, near-death experience
recovering from anaesthetic

+ EFFECTS

helps you come to terms with, or come back to, reality
exerts a grounding influence
focuses and centers
opens you to inspiration, but helps you apply it to the material world
encourages you to make decisions, paying attention to the finer details
promotes a lively interest in the outside world

After a traumatic experience, such as a car crash, people often dissociate themselves (in spirit) from the present. This can be a positive way of coping with acute trauma, but you need to be able to return, and Sundew helps bring you back to the here and now. It may also assist students to concentrate or start new projects. Also consider this essence if you know you are habitually vague and tend to withdraw into yourself — by doing so you may actually be hiding resentment, perhaps because others aren't paying much attention to you; Sundew can help with that feeling.

Hematite <small>(EIRE)</small>

— INDICATIONS
for when you are feeling:
"spacey," uneasy, or vulnerable
downright fearful
have the impression that someone or something is getting at you

+ EFFECTS
brings a feeling of safety
allows you to feel light, but strong
helps pull your energy down into the Earth, and "ground" it

Hematite is a very shiny black stone. In the 1920's there was a fashion for hematite mirrors, because the mineral reflects everything so well. It is said to do the same to any negative vibrations that are directed toward you. Some essence therapists give children who feel especially worried or particularly unsafe in the world little hematite stones to carry in their pockets and hold when needed, and this has been found to be helpful in many cases. The essence works in a similar way to the gem.

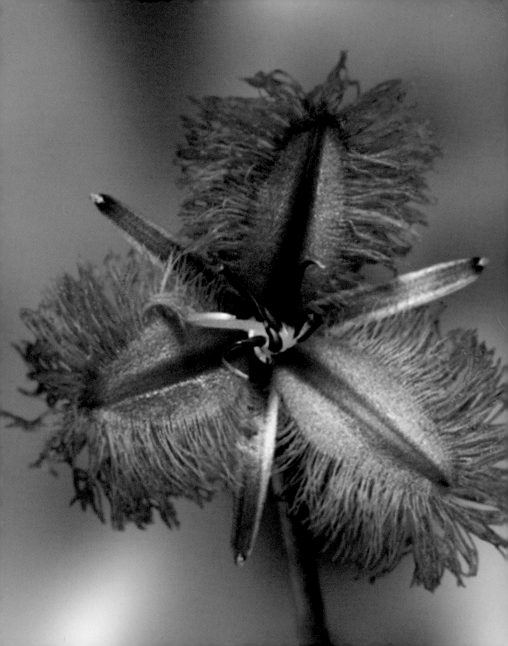

Fringed Violet (AUS)

— INDICATIONS

shock — recent, or long past

need for psychic protection

surgical operations, accidents, birth trauma (for mother and baby)

feeling drained by other people or by certain situations

damaged aura

rebirthing, past-life work, or other deep cathartic emotional experiences

+ EFFECTS

calms the effects of shock

helps you build up effective psychic protection

repairs damage to your aura after severe physical trauma (surgery, accidents), drug taking, or loss of consciousness

Fringed Violet encourages the reintegration of your physical and etheric bodies after a sudden shock or upset, which may have caused them to partially separate (remember the expression "to jump out of your skin with fright"?) Combine it with Angelsword (see page 196) for an extra-powerful protective effect; for a room spray add Boab as well. Fringed Violet treats shock months or even years after the event, and it's never too late to do so. If left unresolved, trauma can be stored in the body and may contribute to the development of many physical illnesses, from eczema to cancer, or mental problems such as a nervous breakdown.

Iona Pennywort (UK)

— INDICATIONS

fear of or fascination with the dark or shadow side of life

dark or demonic thoughts, states of mind, or phobias

psychic fears, superstition

possession by the supernatural or demonic

defying, or breaking, spiritual or karmic laws

+ EFFECTS

releases deep fears or delusions about yourself that are held in the psyche

encourages you to confront and accept the darker side of yourself

brings in the protective light of the Holy Spirit/Source

facilitates self-redemption

engenders scrupulous behavior

discourages judgment of others

This essence is partly about acknowledging and integrating all aspects of yourself, and confronting hidden fears with honesty. When you deny or fear the darker parts of yourself or of life, you create illusion, self-deception and judgment of yourself and other people. Iona Pennywort helps bring light into the darkest corners of the soul, encourages you to realize that darkness coexists with light as part of the whole, and shows you that it's this very dark which throws into relief the brightness of that light.

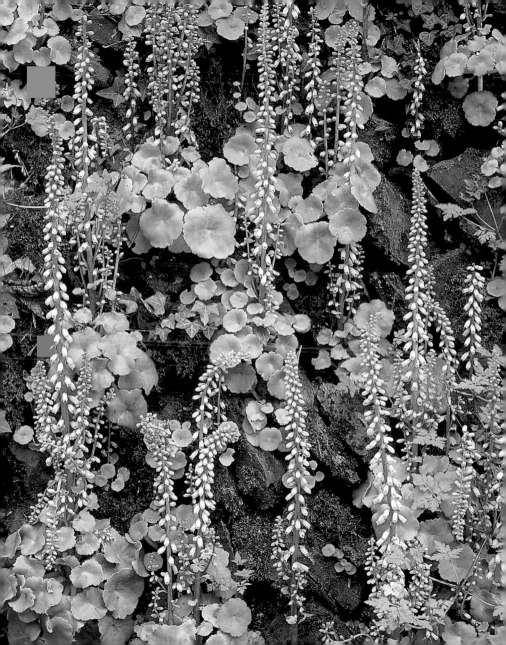

Cell Phone Combination (NLD)

— INDICATIONS
anyone who uses a cell phone
for child and teenage users especially
headache after sustained cell phone use
sensitivity to electricity and electrical devices

+ EFFECTS
provides protection against cell phone radiation
cuts down the stress generated by cell phone use

This combination contains Mycena (mushroom essence) for purification, Terra combination for stress/tension, and Impatiens (the Bloesem variety) for irritation and impatience. It can be used in several ways. When talking on your cell phone, hold CPC in your hand or place the bottle in your pocket, or, each morning, place one or two drops of CPC at the place where the phone rests against your head. If you already have a "cell phone" headache, apply one or two drops to this same place. Note: if you use the phone regularly, it is important to buy a good-quality phone shield. This is especially crucial for children and teenagers, because their neurological systems are still developing and are therefore particularly vulnerable to the problems that cell phone radiation may cause.

Buffalo (USA)

— INDICATIONS

physically or emotionally stressed

out of balance

a busy mind that won't slow down

for healers and practitioners working with distressed clients

+ EFFECTS

provides a secure, deep grounding

slows you down

encourages you to enter the present moment

helps you stay deeply connected to the earth while

you expand spiritually

This essence can help you slow down and become more grounded, and get in touch with the rhythms of the Earth. It is also appropriate when you need to remain anchored in particularly challenging times or difficult situations. The buffalo is sacred in many traditional Native American societies and is the animal that teaches stillness, encouraging inner quiet, calm, and contemplation.

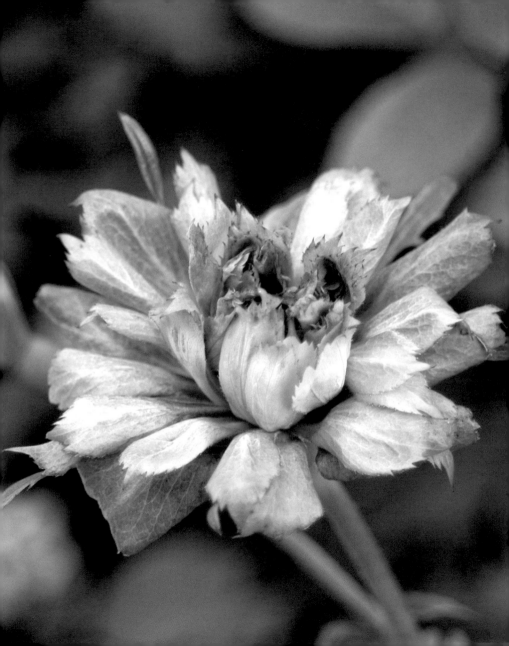

Change

All life is change — a continual stream of endings and beginnings that enables you to develop. First accepting, then adapting to change can initially be destabilizing and exhausting, so it is human to want things to stay the same. Yet resisting change blocks the flow of life, which can lead to problems ranging from low energy and tangible physical disorders to emotional or spiritual distress. Essences help bring about positive change when you are ready, but they encourage, suggest, and support rather than push. If you feel change coming or are in the midst of it, would like support, yet don't see what you need among the essences here, a general combination such as Stuck in a Rut or Soul Support could be helpful instead.

GREEN ROSE

Green Rose *(AUS)*

— INDICATIONS

you keep backsliding on healthy diets and exercise regimes
just cannot complete a change you need to make
those "new leaves" you turn over don't last
suffer from indolence and inertia
begin changes well, but always end up back where you started
may become negative and defensive
blame others for your own lack of progress

+ EFFECTS

strengthens the mind
enables you to focus
ends cycles of defeat
supports you in making a breakthrough
helps you master your inner self-saboteur

Green Rose enhances forward movement out of a phase of stagnation or through a problem, without your suddenly finding yourself back at square one. Helpful for fighting listlessness and the repetition of mistakes, it supports those who are battling against addictive behavior patterns and/or physical substance addictions, from cigarettes and alcohol to hard drugs, and who are becoming frustrated because no matter how hard they feel they try, they keep ending up back where they began.

Peridot (ALASKA)

— INDICATIONS

fear and worry at the beginning of something new
feeling that if you try to change, you will fail
insecurity in the initial phase of any new development

+ EFFECTS

offers support for fresh starts
enhances new growth
encourages you to embrace new experiences
facilitates the incubation of new ideas

Essences made from gems and minerals bring structure and stability, and Peridot is the special gem for new beginnings. Its essence supports you if you are feeling unprotected because what you know and are used to has fallen away, but the new has not yet come in to take its place. It also helps you create — and feel — real, authentic safety, instead of manipulating the situation in order to create an illusion of it.

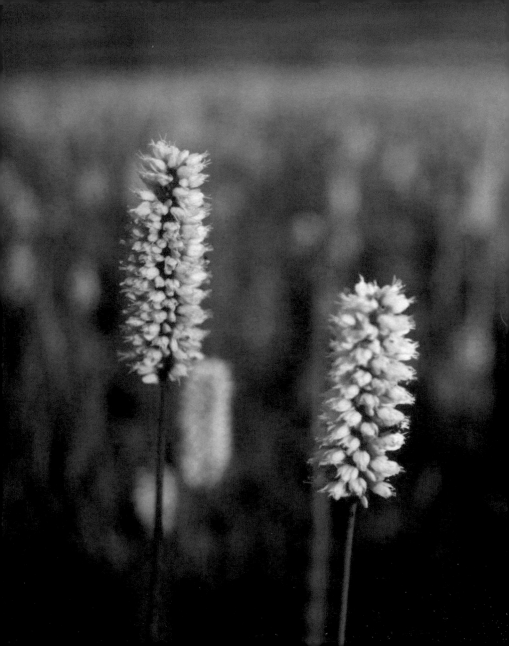

Bistort (UK)

— INDICATIONS
wondering *"Why me?"*
in crisis
feeling threatened and vulnerable during change
tendency to collapse when faced with changes of direction

+ EFFECTS
helps you feel that you are being held up and
strengthened by inner scaffolding
provides loving support for you during change

During any new direction or period of transition, there will be times when you cannot help trying to block the changes taking place (even if it was you who set them in motion), or you may even move into self-destruct mode. Bistort will help support you when this happens. However, it is best to combine it with, or substitute it for, Dog Rose (Bailey type) if you feel that you have gone out on a limb to make these changes and are now wondering whether you have made a big mistake, and/or you fear that your friends disapprove of the initiatives you have taken.

Interesting Times (USA)

— INDICATIONS

facing, or already in the midst of, profound changes
major life shifts in your job, relationships, home, or health
new life phases, like parenthood or menopause
old securities disappearing
challenges to your long-held belief system
issues refusing to be swept under the carpet anymore

+ EFFECTS

enhances your strength and invites courage
soothes fraught nerves and heals pain
acts as a catalyst for positive growth and change

The "upheaval" essence, Interesting Times is very appropriate for the period we are living in. Human and planetary consciousness is shifting, much of what was familiar is starting to be questioned or to fall away, information is appearing that may radically change old beliefs, and we are being faced with moving on in many areas of life — sometimes whether we want to or not. On a higher level, this essence (which contains Red Hollyhock, Valerian, Master Yarrow, Horseradish, and more) can also strengthen and repair your auric shield, for it needs to be resilient and whole to protect you properly in challenging times such as these.

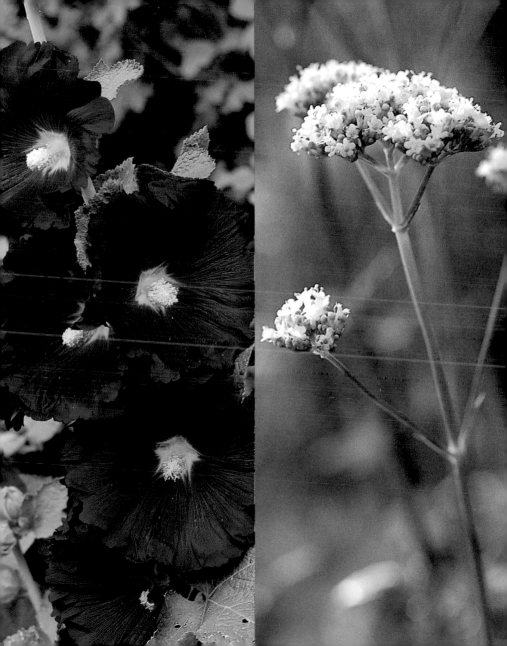

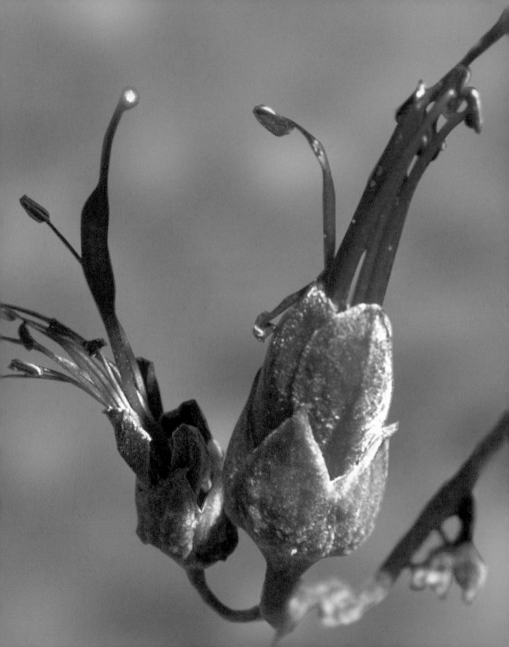

Bauhinia (AUS)

— INDICATIONS

resistance to change of *all* types
resistance to new things in general
reluctance to try new methods of doing things, visit new places or cultures
rigid outlook
uncomfortable with new technology

+ EFFECTS

opens you up to the idea of change being potentially "good"
encourages your interest in its possibilities, even before it occurs
allows you to become more accepting and open-minded
creates a flexible approach to new things

This essence is helpful if you are trying to make positive changes because you know you should, but you're feeling the natural nervousness and resistance many humans feel about anything new (such as becoming net-literate when you are intimidated by computers). Bauhinia allows you to be enthusiastic about, and appreciative of, the new and unfamiliar. However, if the resistance to something new has more of a racial basis, try Slender Rice Flower — the "we are all one" essence.

Black Mushroom (USA)

— INDICATIONS

you feel that everything is changing too fast
are unable to move with the times
it's all too much for you
you may be anxious if away from home for long
have become stuck or bogged down
are resisting leaving an outgrown relationship or
career that is no longer fulfilling

+ EFFECTS

helps you adapt readily to change
enables you to take positive opportunities in your stride
encourages you to feel that you can cope

If the indications above look at all familiar and you feel you would benefit from Black Mushroom, check some additional aspects. Do you also suffer from stiffness? "Can't move" is one of the physical manifestations of feeling unable to go fast enough, or being stuck. Or might you have problems with your neck, back, calves, or ankles? They can suggest the same. If so, it may be a good idea to tackle this on the physical level, too, with a gentle but disciplined activity that encourages flexibility but lets you go at your own pace — such as tai chi, yoga, martial arts, or chi qong.

Beaver *(USA)*

— INDICATIONS
difficulty turning new ideas and thoughts into action and reality

feeling unmotivated

lazy

indecisive

+ EFFECTS
facilitates clear thinking and planning

supports project creation and implementation

encourages problem-solving

boosts efficiency and industriousness

This is a great essence to choose if you are planning to make changes happen, are thinking about new projects, or especially if you want to create a new life for yourself, because Beaver is the master architect and builder. This remedy also helps you accept that structure is a necessary part of the creative process if you want to see your dreams become reality, for even the very best ideas need a solid framework to hold them steady and help them take form in the physical world.

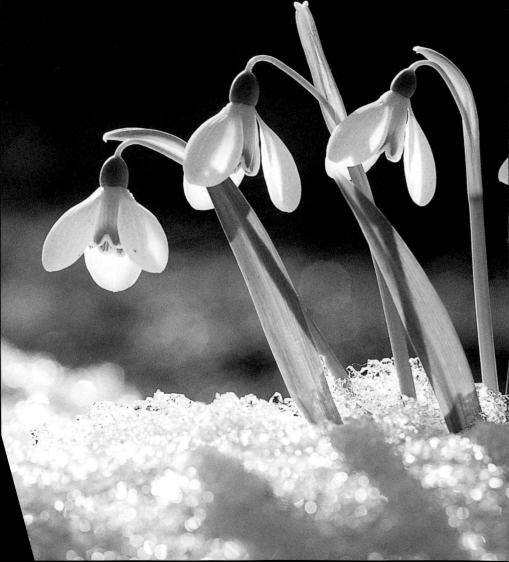

Letting go

Being able to let go of what you no longer need is the key to surviving change. It insures that, when it is time, you can move out of bad situations or stagnation into a far better place, whether in relationships, work, or any other area of your life. Yet this can be very hard because it often feels as if present encumbrances are all that's preventing us from floating away — small wonder most of us fear letting go of the old before the new is in place. These essences can encourage you to trust the process of change with all its challenges and transformative power. They can also help you decide what to leave behind and support you to do it, so that when you're ready, you can move forward with hope, confidence, and enthusiasm — free at last.

SNOWDROP

Snowdrop (UK)

— INDICATIONS

afraid to leave this life
fear of the process of dying
hanging on to life when it is time to let go
grief
the dark night of the soul
negative/destructive attitudes

+ EFFECTS

provides inner strength and encourages peaceful surrender
enables you to yield and let go as a prelude to spiritual rebirth
helps you accept that death leads to liberation, and your soul is eternal
offers transcendence of the physical side of life
brings optimism and hope; alleviates fear

Snowdrop supports those who are preparing for death — the greatest letting-go of all. Along with birth, it is one of the most profound changes for a human being, albeit a positive one, for it is a prelude to rest, healing, renewal, and return. This essence helps someone who is near death to see the light that really is there at the end of the tunnel and to move toward its origin, celebrating the passing of the old and the coming of the new without fear, and facing this new stage calmly and with joy.

Butterfly (USA)

— INDICATIONS

undergoing therapy, facing unresolved wounds
going through any type of emotional healing
changes in your relationships or at work
unwilling to let go
adolescence, menopause, the dying
for babies and young children during key developmental stages
for anyone who feels resistant to change

+ EFFECTS

encourages letting go and moving on
allows you to trust that all will be well
introduces a feeling of lightness and grace
enables you to move forward

This essence encourages a sense of being supported during change
and transition. Besides being used to help those undergoing therapy
of different types, Butterfly is also given to young children who become
unsettled and wake up at night, perhaps having previously been "good"
sleepers. This is especially common during the first two years of life, for
this is a period when several brief but intense phases of neurological
development take place. The remedy is also helpful for little ones when
they are beginning to crawl, or for children experiencing a growth spurt.

Red Henbit *(NLD)*

— INDICATIONS

stuck in chaos
hardly know where to begin to sort it out
for those whose environments need tidying up
too many things to do
difficulty organizing and structuring

+ EFFECTS

helps make tidying up a pleasure
brings clarity to chaos
fosters delight and satisfaction in sorting things out
enables you to focus on your task
promotes energy, vitality, and renewed sexual energy

This essence is great if you are making positive changes by moving home or office, clearing out your workspace, or tidying a chaotic home or workshop to restore order and harmony. Red Henbit is also a catalyst for promoting love of your environment and renewing your vitality, which can become absorbed and dissipated when you are surrounded by disorder or rubbish, for clutter also "holds" stagnant energy like a soggy washcloth holding stale water. It may even attract negativity to a workplace or home: another good reason for the regular clearouts that are the basis of all space-clearing methods (such as feng shui).

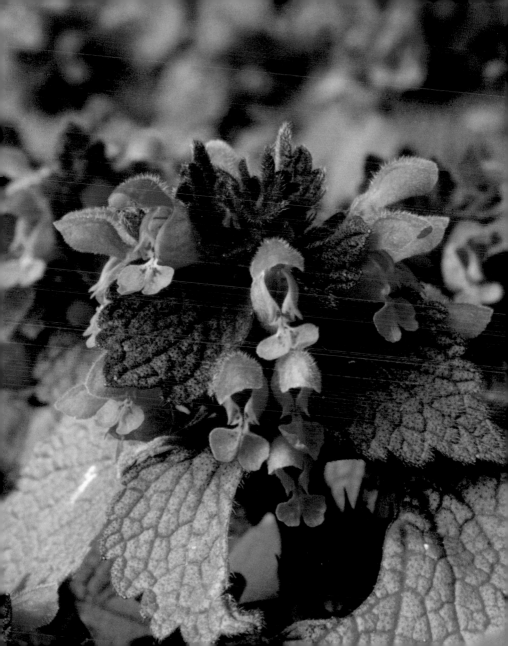

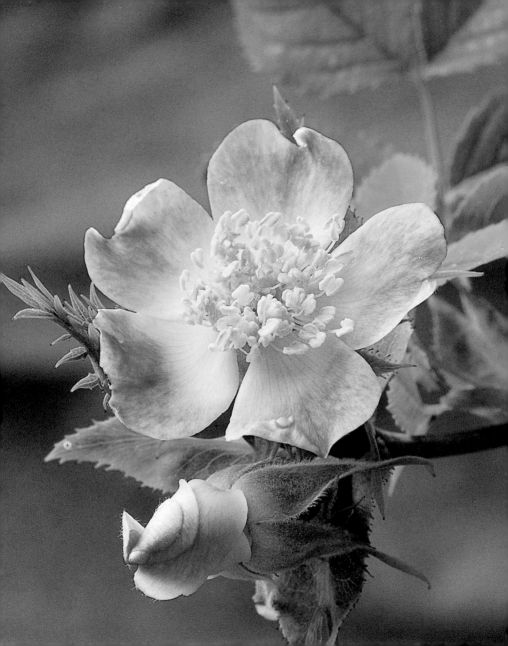

Wild Rose (UK)

— INDICATIONS

not happy, but just don't believe you can change things
resigned to your fate, given up trying to improve things
feel almost paralyzed by apathy
washed out, always tired
make pretty boring company at the moment
feel an underlying hopeless sadness
uncomplaining: you've come to regard the situation as normal

+ EFFECTS

replaces resignation with a sense of purpose
invites you to jump-start the necessary changes yourself
helps get you back in the driving seat of your own life
brings a renewed and lively interest in the world
introduces hope, joy, and determination

This is the remedy for making changes happen yourself, rather than for coping with ones you didn't initiate but are having to manage anyway. It is appropriate if you are not actively miserable, just resigned to your situation ("I've learned to live with it") whether it's an unhappy home life, unsatisfactory job, or chronic illness. Yet Wild Rose shows there's another way, that positive change is possible — and that, in fact, it is you yourself who can bring it about.

Bottlebrush (AUS)

— INDICATIONS

cannot move on
resistant to change
trying to break old bad habits
overwhelmed by major life changes or phases
approaching death

+ EFFECTS

enables you to move on
brushes away the past
helps you go with the necessary flow
enhances your ability to cope
brings calmness and serenity

This essence assists in the calm, assured transition to a new phase, whether it is a new relationship, home, or country, a major new stage in your life (school-leaving, retirement), or a new physical cycle that is beginning or ending (adolescence, pregnancy, parenthood, menopause, old age). Bottlebrush is also used at a physical level for constipation. When combined with Boronia, it can be very effective following relationship breakups if you cannot stop thinking about or pining for that person, nor let go of your time together.

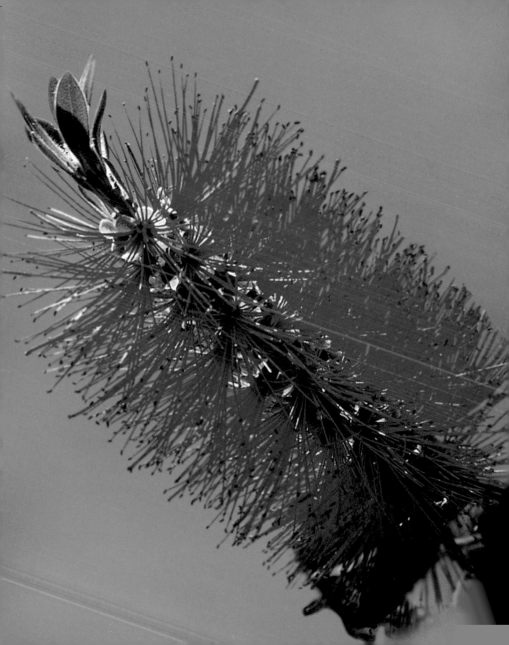

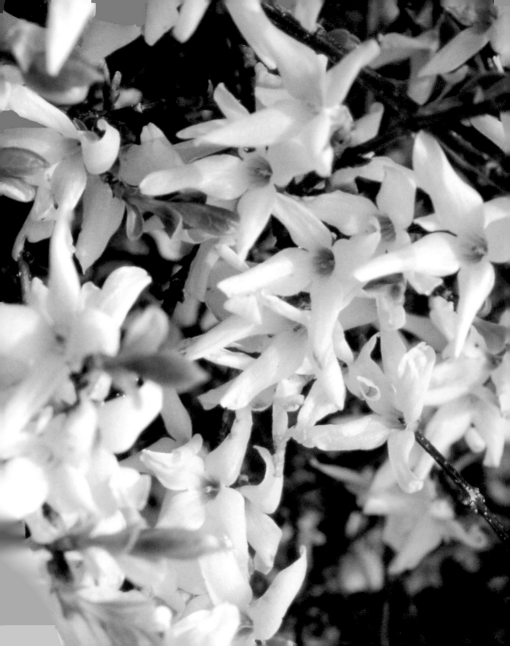

Forsythia (Can)

— INDICATIONS

being stuck in a dysfunctional relationship
repeated problem relationships
addictions to cigarettes, drugs, or alcohol
old habits that no longer serve you
behavior patterns that fill you with self-reproach, even self-loathing
feeling powerless to change any of this

+ EFFECTS

transforms, motivates, acts as a catalyst for change
enables you to respond intuitively with the "right action" for you
supports you in letting go of a dysfunctional relationship
helps with the release of long-held grievances
encourages you to jettison any repetitive negative thoughts

Forsythia is the remedy for addiction — whether physical, mental, or emotional. Herbalists used its yellow flowers to help detoxify the liver, the organ bearing the greatest burden when you are addicted to a substance. The sturdy little branches, on which the flowers are the first sign of new life after winter, are said to represent the strength that will be needed to change old, ingrained patterns. The message that comes with this essence is: *"Allow the golden yellow of my blossoms to bathe you in the light of transformation. Let me strengthen your willingness to move forward."*

Morning Glory *(USA)*

— INDICATIONS

living in the past
dislike of the present
romanticizing days gone by
inability or unwillingness to change a current unpleasant situation

+ EFFECTS

shows you how to use happy past memories as a
springboard for a bright future
encourages you to look forward with enthusiasm
increases your faith in tomorrow — and the day after

Elderly people aren't the only ones who may like to live in the past; people of all ages can do so if the present is not a good time for them. But though happy past times can be comforting and a delight to remember, instead of being used as a burrow to hide your head in, they can also be made into steps on the life ladder which can help you climb upward to better days. Morning Glory can support anyone who feels that their past was a golden age and frankly prefers to live there rather than in the present, because this essence encourages renewed faith in yourself and a positive, progressive attitude toward the future.

Blue China Orchid (AUS)

— INDICATIONS

insufficient willpower to make changes

addicted to certain people, substances, or ways of behaving

battling against obsessive behavior patterns

not strong

unwilling to give up old, negative ways

+ EFFECTS

breaks the hold of old patterns

introduces self-control and discipline

strengthens the will

helps offer direction

supports you in making positive change

This is the essence for strengthening the will and taking back control of the self. It can help you break ingrained habits (which, like lumpy old armchairs, you still have to fight against sinking back into) and to overcome your own former programming to insure that you don't start using them again — even though you know those habits erode your quality of life. Blue China Orchid can also be used for children who have become set in certain negative patterns such as night-waking, crying, being destructive and "naughty" to get attention, or reacting instantly and powerfully if they don't get their own way.

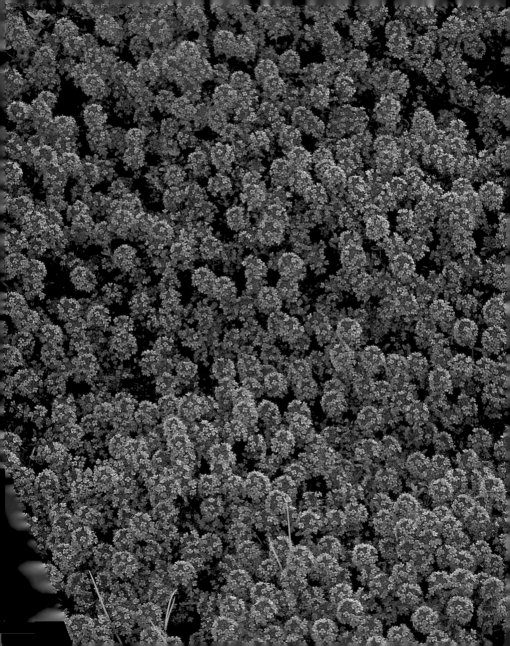

Intuition

Your intuition is the most powerful ally you
have. It sees around life's corners, through its
smokescreens, and penetrates straight to the
heart of the most complex problems, whispering
"this way" in your inner ear. Said to be your
higher spiritual self talking — that part which is
connected directly to the Source (God, Buddha,
the Divine) — it's the part of you that cannot be
fooled, the part that's always right, the part that
just knows. Yet you cannot always hear that wise
inner voice clearly through the static of everyday
life, and don't always trust it when you do. The
following essences help to clear the mind and
sharpen the intuition, so that you can find your
way forward when you are unable to see the
wood for the trees.

Clarity (INDIA)

— INDICATIONS

lack of direction in life

poor focus

lack of self-awareness

isolation, alienation, disconnection from the rest of the world

cannot concentrate

excess sexual energy

+ EFFECTS

enhances clarity of thought

deepens awareness and wisdom

promotes clairvoyance

develops your intuition and the ability to see to the heart of things

helps you meditate deeply

At a higher level, this essence helps you align yourself with your soul's purpose here on Earth, and enhances your sense of being a spiritual being in a physical body. At a more physical level, Clarity (which contains Thyme and Parochetus) may also be helpful to teenagers (boys especially) whose sexuality is rising, but who are also having to concentrate on an increasingly demanding academic workload and focus on exams at school or college.

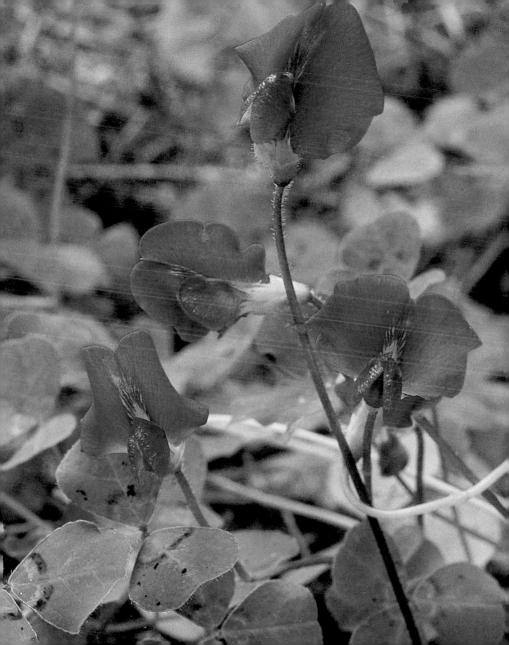

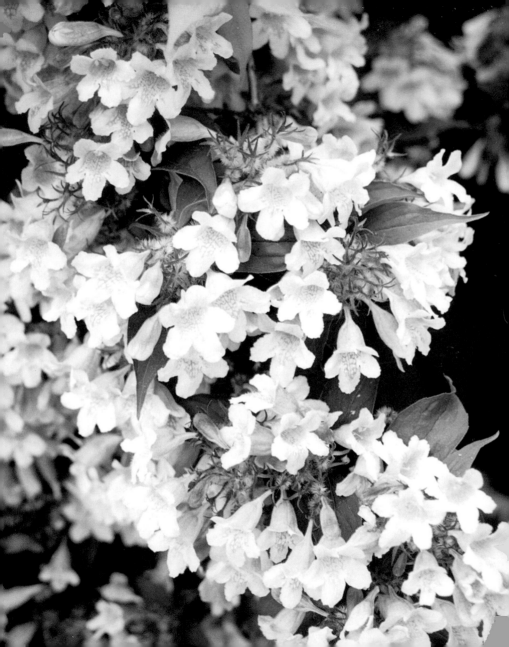

Weigela (CAN)

— INDICATIONS

you do not understand the lessons life keeps presenting you with
your life isn't making any sense
you are not learning from the things that happen to you

+ EFFECTS

brings realization of what each experience is really teaching you
encourages you to grow and develop, even when times are hard
shows you how to learn from the lessons life offers you
helps you see others as your teachers

The "teaching" essence, Weigela can be especially useful when you apparently have an "accident," or experience physical or emotional traumas that seem to come from nowhere. This remedy also helps you understand that both your self and your behavior are mirrored back to you by those you meet — often by people you don't even like, or whose actions you find objectionable. This happens so that you can see those particular aspects of yourself reflected in them, and thereby come to understand yourself better.

Mauve Mullein *(USA)*

— INDICATIONS
unable to receive spiritual information
difficulty accessing spiritual guidance

+ EFFECTS
brings patience and understanding
enhances your intuition and inner knowing
helps develop your third eye
strengthens your connection to higher wisdom

This essence encourages the healthy, balanced development and functioning of the sixth (third eye) and seventh (crown) chakras. The sixth chakra is indigo/purple, the color of the mauve mullein flower, and the seat of your intuition — perhaps that's why "inner knowing" is nicknamed the sixth sense. The seventh chakra, color violet, is the one through which you make a personal and direct connection with divine energy, by whichever name you wish to call it: God, the Universal Source of Love and Light, Buddha. Mauve Mullein also helps you link in with the collective consciousness (the network of human and spiritual awareness that spans our planet — and which some say links the entire Universe), so that "Out There" also becomes "In Here."

Owl *(USA)*

— INDICATIONS

difficulty making decisions

confused

cannot decide what's true — not only for others, but also for you

unable to see what lies beneath the surface of an issue

understanding is limited by your own beliefs

+ EFFECTS

helps you "see clearly in the darkness"

highlights things that need your attention and helps you face them

brings mental clarity

enables you to see the truth of a situation very clearly

enhances your intuition

puts you in touch with higher wisdom for help and guidance

This is an essence for the times in your life when you have a feeling that something's not right, but you cannot see what it is, or where. Owl will help you when you are attempting to find a way forward through a confusing situation, and trying to clear your mind.

Alder (ALASKA)

— INDICATIONS
taking life at surface value
unclear inner vision — feeling muddled, muddied
unable to respond to life lessons appropriately

+ EFFECTS
enables you to respond quickly to new learning opportunities
helps you perceive the truth
brings clarity of vision

The "clear seeing" remedy, Alder helps you access information that is outside your usual range of perception. It also encourages you to understand each learning opportunity (frequently offered in the form of a challenge, problem, or difficulty) as it is given to you in life, and to be able to respond to it in the most appropriate way — a way that will help you in your development. If you are feeling muddled but also "separate, and out of touch," consider also using the gem essence Moldavite from the same range as Alder.

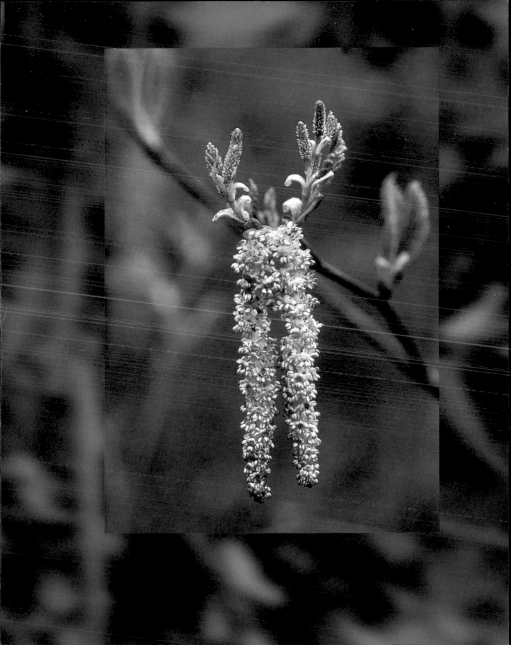

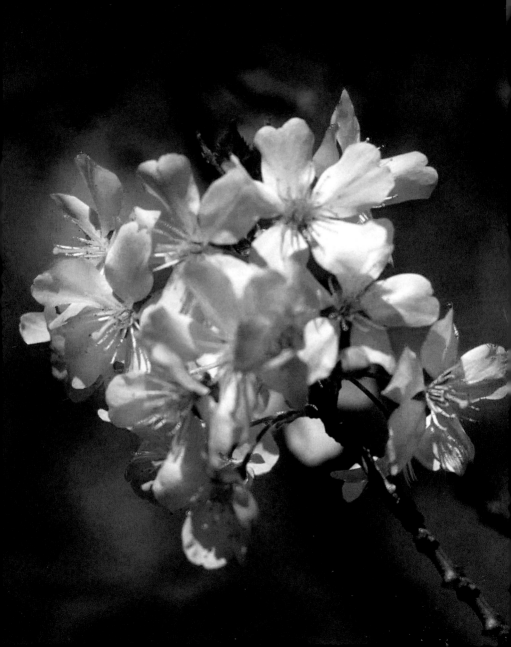

Almond (UK)

— INDICATIONS
you feel the need for a guide in your life
find moving on to a new path alarming
have become enmeshed in old patterns but can't see how they arose
are unsure what is your own true intuition talking, and what isn't
cannot see your way ahead

+ EFFECTS
awakens the "teacher" inside you
empowers you to hear, and believe, your own intuition
brings increasing insight
liberates you from old patterns that have had you dancing to their tune

Almond is a gentle essence but one that is very deep. It shows you that everything you ever need, including trustworthy guidance, can be found right here, inside your own self. It offers support, reassurance, and comfort if you are going in a new direction, and teaches you to rely on and trust your own intuition. In addition, Almond helps you discover true self-confidence, so that you are able to remain unbothered by any opposition from others who feel threatened by the changes in you.

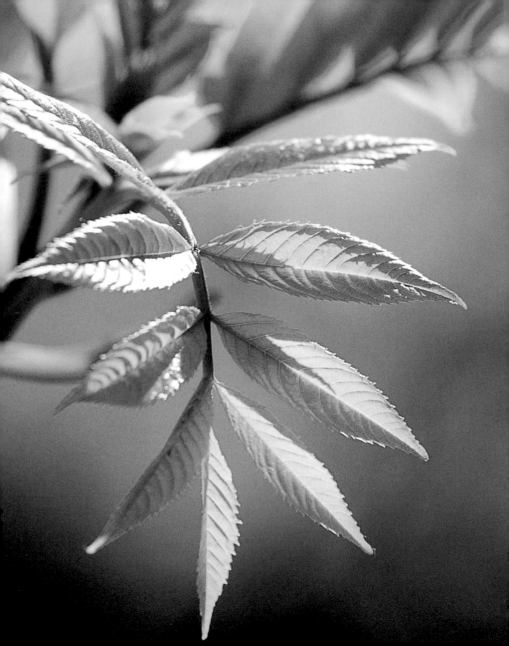

Spiritual development

Spiritual development has many aspects — and increasing sensitivity to things that are as real as you are but cannot be seen or touched is just one of them. It is also of paramount importance to stay safe, grounded, and take it gently while your consciousness expands, so that you don't develop too fast or become too "fey," but instead can integrate your growing awareness into ordinary life in a balanced way. All the following essences can help increase psychic and intuitive abilities, but each also offers something extra that you may find welcome on a spiritual journey.

Reunion *(UK)*

— INDICATIONS

fearful of your expanding consciousness
concerned as you become increasingly sensitive
unsettled by multidimensional awareness
cannot integrate or ground your new expanded perception

+ EFFECTS

eases your fear of any new shifts of perception
grounds and integrates your awareness that life is multidimensional
integrates your right- and left-brain perspectives

Reunion was made from a twin ash (*Fraxinus excelsior*). The ash tree was sacred to many past cultures including that of the Celts, who believed it linked the past, present, and future, its "keys" (seedpods) symbolizing the understanding of how all things are connected. In Norse mythology, too, Odin used the ash tree to gain the secrets of runes and enlightenment. Today, the essence made from the twin ash is a reassuring and stabilizing one for the stage of evolution that both humankind and the planet have now reached — especially because the consciousness of many people is developing rapidly at present.

Crow (USA)

— INDICATIONS
feel a spiritual calling but are uncertain how, or whether, to follow it
for those who see the physical and spiritual worlds as separate

+ EFFECTS
for developing a shamanic view and understanding of reality
helps you see beyond the everyday world
supports the development and acknowledgment of your intuition
enhances your shamanic power

Crow is the essence for aspiring shamans, and for those who would like to develop the shamanic way of looking at reality. This is that everything is alive, everything is animate, and that it isn't only humans who are sentient; streams, rocks, mountains, forests, plants, and animals are, too. Shamanism teaches that the spirit world is just as real as the physical world that you can touch with your fingers and see with your eyes — and the implications of this are huge.

Bush Iris (AUS)

— INDICATIONS

atheism

overly materialistic

for those losing their former spiritual belief or faith

being afraid of dying

+ EFFECTS

fosters faith, and a sense of being supported spiritually

awakens spirituality

encourages the opening of the third-eye chakra, seat of

intuition and perception

enhances spiritual awareness

supports and brings reassurance to those close to death

Bush Iris encourages you to be aware that there is more to existence than the things your usual five senses can detect, and supports the development of your intuition. If given to those near death, especially if they are fearful of passing over, Bush Iris can help bring about a calm, peaceful transition. It may also reduce the need for painkilling drugs when someone is dying, leaving their awareness and perception of the spiritual help that comes to them at this time (to guide them to the light) clearer and unclouded, the better to draw comfort and reassurance from it.

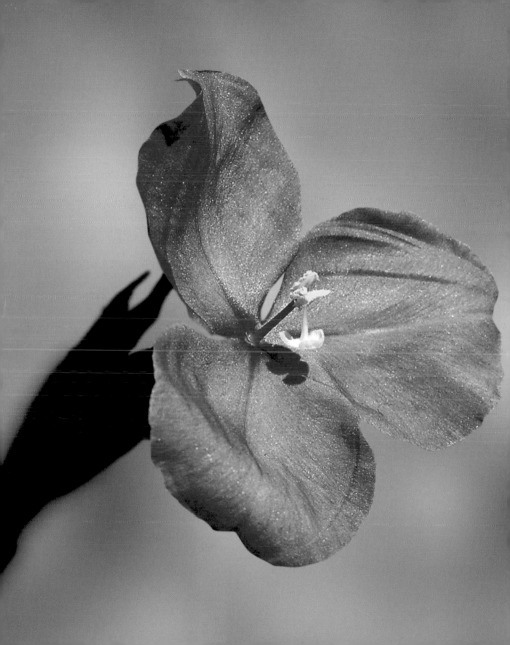

Whale (CAN)

— INDICATIONS

alienation: not feeling part of the whole web of life

problems understanding that there is more to existence than the physical

ethnocentricity: feeling your own group is superior

arrogance — of all types

+ EFFECTS

amplifies your capacity to sense energy

enhances your ability to transmit energy with your hands

allows you to hear more subtle sounds, even in the inner city

helps you receive and interpret information about your origins and path

facilitates telepathy and clairsentience

acts as a good general physical tonic

This is an essence of choice for all healers. The message that came with it when it was first made is: "*I am the giant of the sea. When you want to know what you are really capable of, come to me.*"

Star Sapphire *(ALASKA)*

— INDICATIONS

worrying over small details of your spiritual progress
difficulty making the right choices or right connections in your life
cannot tune in to spiritual information about your purpose on this earth
doubt and uncertainty about your path in life
difficulty trusting the Universe

+ EFFECTS

enables you to trust fully in the Universe
helps manifest your destiny
encourages you to focus on what your soul needs in order to progress
allows you to get more done

Star Sapphire highlights the importance of trust in spiritual development — trusting the Universe to guide you in the direction you need to go. This is not easy and it may take years, but the relief when you do reach that stage can be enormous, for the weight of worry and doubt you may have been carrying for so long simply lifts. When this happens, you often find that you have more energy, too, because the vitality that was formerly sapped by carrying your burden of fear and uncertainty has returned. Star Sapphire is also appropriate if you find you are overly concerned with your spiritual progress, as worrying about this may absorb a lot of energy and result in your becoming inward-looking.

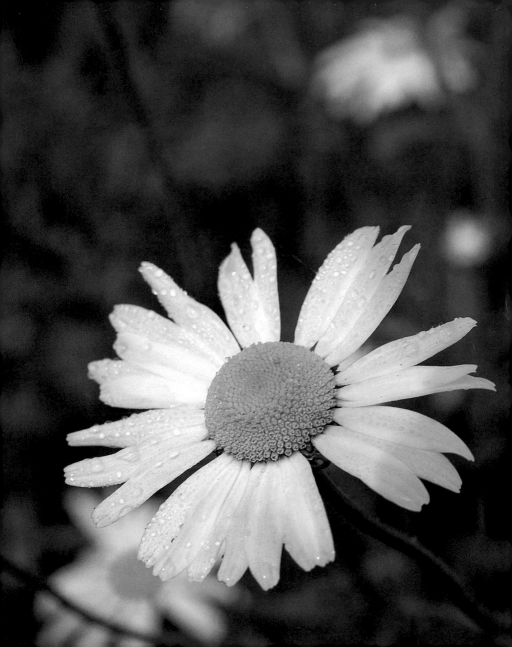

Ox Eye Daisy *(CAN)*

— INDICATIONS

focusing too hard on one thing
having a narrow perspective
being fearful of seeing too clearly
needing a new angle on an old problem

+ EFFECTS

produces synthesis and alchemy — can put things together in a new way
enables you to see the bigger picture
encourages you to regard old issues or problems in a new light
helps you see things clearly

This essence is the remedy for vision or the visionary, and it works on several different levels. Physically, it is said to affect the eyes and ears, and may help you develop better eyesight. At an emotional level, it is a remedy of choice when you are struggling to "see" something in a brand new way. It also relates to the kidney meridian of traditional Chinese medicine — blockages in this pathway are associated with fear, an emotion that may hold you back from looking at problems in a fresh way, but which this essence can help release. Spiritually, the essence supports the third-eye (brow) chakra, seat of intuition and perception.

Chestnut *(S AF)*

− INDICATIONS

having trouble visualizing things when you meditate

expanding spiritually but without enough grounding or protection

feeling trapped or alienated in your physical life

+ EFFECTS

enhances visualization and aids meditation

supports safe psychic development

exerts a grounding and protective influence

enables you to contact helpers from higher dimensions, such as angels

facilitates the gentle, harmonious opening of your third eye — the

seat of intuition, and seeing beyond the physical

Chestnut supports those seeking to develop their psychic abilities, because it helps protect and ground you as well as encouraging a growing spiritual sensitivity: a vital combination of awareness-enhancement and "keeping safe." This is important, because it is fairly common for people who are developing spiritually (like trainee healers) to find that they are rapidly becoming more sensitive, but are not, at first, always able to protect themselves well enough from some of the results.

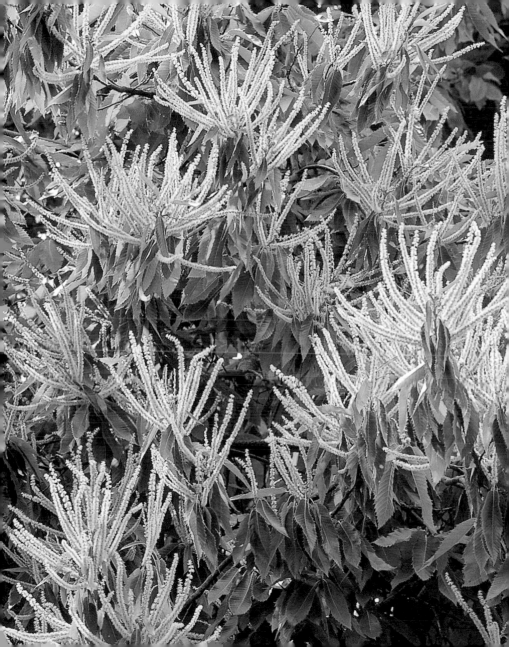

Ararybá (BRA)

— INDICATIONS
difficulty seeing the bigger picture
oversusceptibility to group behavior and pressure
your own boundaries are not strong
you feel vulnerable and unprotected
you have no sense of your own life's purpose

+ EFFECTS
enables you to see things globally
supports telepathic ability
helps you connect with your Higher Self for guidance and support
stimulates an awareness of your soul's mission on the planet, and
strengthens your determination to achieve this
affirms your personal sense of identity
offers protection, and helps heal any gaps in your aura

Ararybá can help show you how we are all linked, both to each other and to the rest of the planet, and how to access your own spiritual support and advice system. It also encourages a sense of the plan behind the "big picture" of existence. One effect of this is that it helps people understand that while human beings are an important part of that big picture or pattern of life, as is everything on earth, we are not the centerpiece around which that pattern is designed.

Mugwort *(USA)*

— INDICATIONS

wondering if there is more to life than this

life just consists of "getting up, eating, working, then going to bed again"

existence seems two-dimensional

you feel cut off from spiritual help

+ EFFECTS

helps develop your psychic skills

facilitates integration of your spiritual learning into everyday life

encourages you to be fully receptive to spiritual information

enables you to go with the flow of any challenges

The "Is this all there is?" essence, Mugwort can also be a potent catalyst for developing psychic awareness and abilities, so it is important to have strong, secure energy-field boundaries before using it. If you feel that perhaps you don't have these yet, first work to strengthen them before taking this essence. There are several good all-round grounding and protective essence combinations that can help here. Have a look at the suggestions and descriptions on pages 208–223 and see if any of them strikes a chord. Also consider contacting a reputable healer or esoteric teacher for additional advice on safe spiritual development and boundary-strengthening.

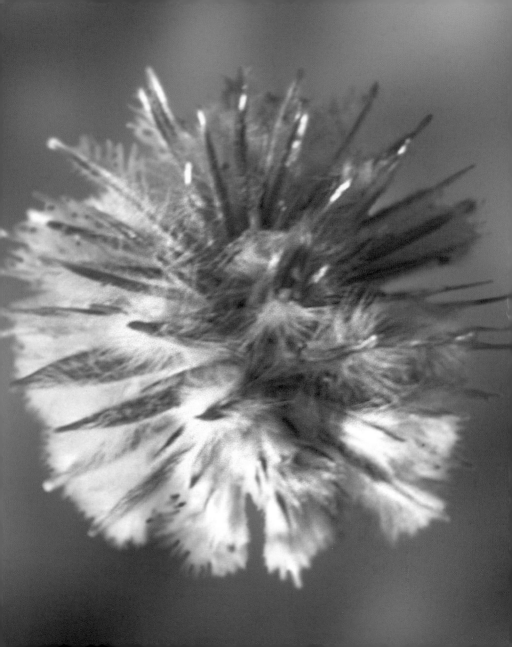

Emergencies

Essences are gentle and subtle, with nothing in them that ordinary science can find except brandy and water, and it usually takes a week or two for their effects to be felt, but several can be used as emergency remedies in acute "need help now" situations. Rescue Remedy is still the best known, but there are many more that can be both fast-acting and highly effective for specific emergencies such as pain, burns, terror, or hysteria, and others that are much used for more minor problems like cuts, bruising, irritability, and sunburn. Here is a selection of some of the best emergency essence remedies to keep in the medicine chest at home, marked with a * if they are also recommended for use at work.

Mulla Mulla

First Aid

Burns
Fireweed (used in the University of São Paulo Hospital burns unit) can be taken internally for mild to severe burns, and/or diluted in water for washing minor burns at home. It is reported to reduce pain effectively and speed healing.

Pimples, boils, and bruises
Angelsword seems to speed healing, too, soothing pain and visibly reducing inflammation from scrapes, minor burns, small boils, pimples, and abscesses. Add three to five drops to two cups of cool water for soothing painful grazes; apply topically and undiluted to bruises to help them resolve faster and hurt less. Some users report that Angelsword, dabbed onto a burgeoning spot, works better than regular acne creams.

Sunburn and radiation
Mulla Mulla is also used for burns including sunburn (try Solaris, too, if you've been in the sun too long). When Mulla Mulla is given to people undergoing radiation therapy, it is reported to reduce the amount of burning they experience from the treatment. It should be taken immediately before a session, as well as morning and night for the duration of the course. Essence therapists also suggest this remedy for burning sensations *anywhere* in the body, including vaginitis, cystitis, and eczema. Taking it orally, or as seven to ten drops added to a warm bath, can help reduce discomfort right away.

Cross and irritable?
You need to try *Impatiens, which can often calm babies, toddlers, older children, and adults immediately. Two or three doses 15–20 minutes apart can be especially effective.

Nearing the end of your strength
If you are very tired but have to keep going, try *Oak as it can give you a new lease on life, and the energy to complete what you are doing — which might be anything from an arduous sponsored walk to childbirth. For the office, consider *Dynamis spray to renew your energy and enthusiasm.

Fear

If you are nervous and shy but have an important interview, social occasion, or work presentation coming up, even one dose of *Crowea or Confid Essence just beforehand can help dissolve your nerves. However, if you are more scared than worried before a forthcoming traumatic event like surgery — or even the relatives from hell coming to visit — Pre-Trauma can be a great stabilizer.

In pain

Aching with arthritis or rheumatism, or suffering from back or joint pain? Pain Cream (used in state hospitals and clinics all over Australia) can be immensely comforting either to rub onto affected areas or as part of a gentle massage. Body Sports lotion is widely used for the relief of sports injury soft-tissue damage and pain.

Constipation

This complaint has been known to respond rapidly to a gemstone essence called Bloodstone: sometimes right there on the massage couch, so the client has had to exit fast...

Herpes

Many people report that dabbing a herpes blister as it is starting, with Spinifex, aborts the attack. It is also said to be effective for cutting, stinging pain such as a clean incision (like a paper cut) with no flesh missing.

In a crisis

When a child or teenager appears suicidal or parasuicidal and you fear for them, try to encourage them to take The Works, especially if they have literally locked themselves in their room and won't come out. This combination essence can stabilize them quickly, so that they will at least allow someone to talk to them. For an adult who is in utter despair, offer Waratah.

Pets and other animals

Rescue animals, those brought in from the wild, animals that have spent a long time isolated in pet stores, and those that are very agitated, frightened, or aggressive can benefit greatly from Animal Care. For immediate help, give two to four drops in water or on a bit of food. If the animal won't take it or come near you, spray it around them.

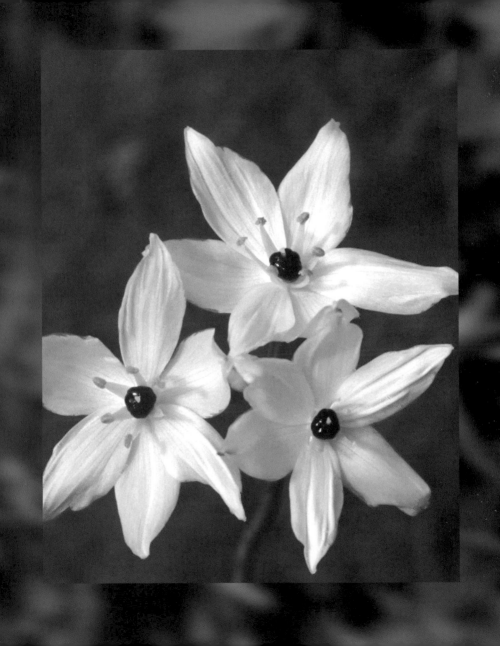

Emergency Combination Power

An emergency essence combination is a must for every handbag, household, school, and office as the essences from which they are made complement each other powerfully. An emergency remedy will start working at once to address the following issues simultaneously.

Feeling safe and calming down

All emergency combinations combat overwhelm, soothe fear, calm terror.

Grounding

"It's as if the ground had disappeared from under my feet." You need grounding after a shock, accident, or trauma, to help renew the "roots" that keep you in contact with the Earth.

Coming back

"I was beside myself" and *"I jumped out of my skin"* are no mere phrases. They illustrate what often happens when you experience sudden severe stress, are very scared, or are deeply shocked — your spirit may instinctively "check out" of your body for a while as a means of coping. While this can be a positive way of protecting yourself from the distress of an extreme situation, such as a car crash, it is important to be able to come back again once it is safe.

Protection and support

"I feel exhausted and spaced out." After trauma, you are vulnerable to negative influences for a while. This can be because it throws you temporarily into a negative state, and like attracts like. It may also be that severe shock or injury can damage your aura, leaving you wide open. Emergency combinations contain powerfully protective essences, plus others to support, rebuild, and strengthen your natural safety barriers.

Great combinations to try:

Emergency Essence
Soul Support
Shock & Trauma
Rescue Remedy
Animals to the Rescue
Animal Care (especially for animals)
Peace in a Storm
First Aid
Crisis Relief

Index of symptoms

From the list below, select the symptom(s) for which you would like an essence or the subject that interests you, then turn to the indicated page(s) for an essence or essences with full description.

existential distress 163
expanding consciousness, fear of 264
exposed, feeling 210
expressing feelings, difficulty in 80, 121

failure, fear of 52
fainting 216
faith, loss of 92, 102, 266
falling apart, sense of 44
false personae 69
fantasizing 214
fatalism 96, 243
fathering 122, 154, 159, 165, 185, 186
fatherless children 177
fatigue see exhaustion; tiredness
fear/fearfulness 23, 49, 63, 69, 91, 217, 220,
    227, 279, 281
fertility problems 39, 102, 105, 111, 127,
    143
fickleness 162
fluid retention 105
focus, lacking 216, 252
forthrightness 149
fostered children 180
frigidity 135, 136
frustration 106, 159, 173, 178, 201
fulfillment, lack of 190, 234
fun see sense of fun, loss of

genitals, dislike of 139
giving up on projects 22, 39, 92, 226
gloom 73, 88
goal-orientation 119, 174
grazes 278
grief 72, 79, 84, 91, 238
grounding 162, 209, 213, 214, 216, 223, 264,
    272, 281
growth spurts 174, 239
grubby, feeling 199
grumpiness 88
guidance, needing 261

hair-tugging 24
hangovers 199
"harmful" external influences, fear of 215
harmful substances, exposure to 205
healers 155, 223
healing energy, resistance to 43
heart, closed 147
heart chakra 10, 83, 137, 145
heart surgery 149, 165
heaviness of spirit 73
helping others see caring; nurturing
helplessness 89
herpes 279
hesitancy 52
Higher Self, connection to 274
homosexuality 118
hopelessness/despairing 49, 91, 92, 95, 243, 279
hormonal imbalance 105, 109, 111
humiliation, fear of 55
humility 68
humor see sense of fun, loss of
"hurt givers" 159
hypersensitivity 23
hypervigilance 27

immunity, low 39, 205
impatience 32, 38, 109, 222
impotence 39, 125, 135, 143
impurity, sense of 197
inadequacy 125
inconsiderateness 152
indecisiveness 53, 235, 257, 269
indolence/laziness 80, 127, 226, 235
inertia 226
infections, trauma from 44
inferiority, feelings of 64, 68
infertility see fertility problems
inflammation 205
injuries, physical 44, 106
insecurity 23, 125, 162, 171, 217, 227
insignificance, feelings of 57

soft touch, seen as 22
space-clearing 91, 207, 213, 240
"spacy" feeling 217
speech difficulties 67, 169, 178
spiritual development/progress 83, 196, 197,
    263-75
spiritual information 256, 258
spiritual protection 209-23
spite 159
spontaneity, lack of 75
sport 127
stagnation 80, 142, 143, 205, 226
stiffness 234
stress 28, 29, 31, 32, 49, 180, 185, 186, 223, 281
stress-related habits 24
striving 28, 31, 32, 126
stubbornness 125
stuttering 169
submissiveness/subservience 89, 103
suffering, others' 63, 189, 193
suicidal feelings 163, 165, 279
sunburn 278
superiority 68
supernatural possession 220
superstition 220
Superwoman 111
suppressed emotions 72, 79
surgery, trauma from 44, 106, 149, 219

tantrums, toddler 173
tasks, completion of 22, 92, 226
teenagers see adolescence
telepathy 102, 274
tension 23, 24, 27, 29, 91, 201
therapy 207, 239
third eye 10, 255, 266, 271, 272
throat chakra 10, 11, 67, 72
tidying up 240
timidity 55, 80
tiredness 8, 22, 37-49, 180, 184, 213, 243, 278
toddlers 173, 278

toxins 201, 205
trauma 44, 106, 216, 255; see also birth trauma
tyranny 118

uncomfortableness 92
undervalued, feeling 181
unfulfilled desire 136
unhappiness see sadness
unloved, feeling 112, 136
unmotivated, feeling 235
unsettled, feeling 171
unwanted, feeling 136
unwholesome lifestyle 205
"upheavals," facing 230
upset 91
uterus prolapse 115

vaginitis 278
vagueness 216
visualization 209, 272
vitality, lack of 24, 38, 49, 61, 127
vulnerability 89, 155, 166, 177, 210, 215, 217,
    229, 274

weakness 49, 60, 205; see also vulnerability
willpower, lack of 247, 248, 249
work/workaholics 28, 31, 38, 111, 146, 174, 184,
    197, 234, 252
worrying 27, 29, 31, 32, 93, 95, 227

zest for life, lack of 76

Index of essences

Essence ranges and their developers

Alaskan Flower Essences

Alaskan Flower Essence Project

PO Box 1369

Homer

Alaska 99603

USA

tel: 1 800 545 3909 (US/Canada)

907 235 2188 (worldwide)

email: info@alaskanessences.com

website: www.alaskanessences.com

*Essences, sprays, and books, plus courses
and seminars: training to practitioner level
worldwide.*

Steve Johnson was a firefighter in the
western United States and Alaska until
health challenges led him to the Bach
remedies. In 1983 the pristine Alaskan
countryside inspired him to begin
preparing essences from its plants,
gems, natural environments, and
weather conditions. He founded the
Alaskan Flower Essence Project in 1984
and continues to research the remedies
(now over 200) with therapist Jane Bell.
Steve also runs an international
practitioner training program and
teaches all over the world.

Araretama Rainforest Essences

Araretama Essencias Naturais Ltda

São Paulo/SP

Brazil

tel: 55 (11) 5531 9068

website: www.araretama.com.br

email: araretama@uol.com.br

*Essences, books, and seminars. Website
version available in English.*

Araretama means "place from which
light arises." These essences, made
from the exotic bromeliads, roots, and
lichens of Brazil's Atlantic rainforests,
were created by Sandra Epstein while
she was researching a cure for a friend's
illness. Sandra's professional background
is in art, therapy, and holistic healing,
which have contributed to her present
work as an essence therapist and healer.
She also teaches around the world.

Australian Bush Flower Essences

45 Booralie Road, Terrey Hills

NSW 2084

Australia

tel: 61 (0) 294 501 388

email: info@ausflowers.com.au

website: www.ausflowers.com.au

Essences, books, creams, sprays and flower cards, videos, and a journals. Training courses (correspondence/live) and seminars training to practitioner level worldwide.

There are more than 90 essences and combinations made from plants and sacred sites in this range developed by Ian White, a fifth-generation Australian herbalist. He practiced naturopathy and homeopathy for over 20 years, and has long pioneered the remedial qualities of Australia's bush plants. These essences are increasingly widely available inter-nationally in health stores, and Ian runs training seminars in Europe, North and South America, Asia, and Australia.

Bach Flower Remedies at:
Healing Herbs Ltd
PO Box 65, Hereford HR2 06X
England
tel: 44 (0) 1873 890218
email: info@healingherbs.co.uk
website: www.healingherbs.co.uk

Healing Herbs' version of the 38 Bach Flower Remedies, stays meticulously faithful to the traditional essence production methods of Dr. Bach. Also wide selections of essence books and herbal products, together with essence consultations, training courses,

seminars, and a practitioner mentoring service.

Dr. Edward Bach Centre
Mount Vernon
Bakers Lane
Sotwell
Oxfordshire OX10 OPZ
England
tel: 44 (0) 491 834678
email: kathy@bachcentre.com
website: www.bachcentre.com

Training courses to practitioner level, Bach Flower Remedies, books, videos and flower cards. Now taken over by the well-known homeopathic products company Nelsons.

Dr. Edward Bach was a remarkable and visionary physician with a busy practice in London's prestigious Harley Street in the 1920's, when his dissatisfaction with modern medicine led him to create the first modern vibrational plant essences — which he named the Bach Flower Remedies. Julian Barnard studied these at the Bach Centre in Oxford, England, and has written several books on the subject. His company, Healing Herbs, is dedicated to maintaining the purity and quality of the original 38 remedies that were developed by Dr. Bach.

Bailey Flower Essences

7 Nelson Road
Ilkley, West Yorkshire LS29 7HN
England
tel: 44 (0) 1943 432012
email: office@baileyessences.com
website: www.baileyessences.com

Essences, books, courses, plus an essence-choosing/checking service using a clipping of the customer's hair and dowsing tuition.

Dr. Arthur Bailey was Senior Lecturer in Electrical and Electronic Engineering at Bradford University in Yorkshire, England, when he became interested in dowsing, conducting rigorous scientific research into the phenomenon. He came across homeopathy and Bach remedies while recovering from ME, then found he could heal by laying on hands. In 1968 he began developing his own remedies from the plants in his Yorkshire garden, which are now sold all over the world.

Findhorn Flower Essences

Cullerne House, Findhorn,
Forres, Moray
Scotland IV36 31YY
tel: 44 (0) 1309 690129
email: info@findhornessences.com
website: www.findhornessences.com

Essences, books, workshops, and training to practitioner level.

Findhorn is a long-established spiritual community in Scotland, whose magical gardens are world famous. This essence range was developed by Marion Leigh, an Australian homoeopath, practitioner, and teacher of esoteric healing. She runs courses to practitioner level at Findhorn, and teaches others around the world.

Flower Essences of Fox Mountain

PO Box 381, Worthington
MA 0198-0381, USA
tel: 1 413 238 4291
email: foxmountain@earthlink.net
www.floweressencesoffoxmountain.com

Essences and booklet.

Kathrin Woodlyn Bateman knew by the age of 11 that she would be a healer, and began studying and using herbs from then on. She began making flower essences in 1989, while also raising two young children and running a farm. Her company grew as her essences were shared from healer to healer, and the range now offers 375. Fox Mountain remedies are used in many countries, although the company remains small.

Flower Essences of the Netherlands
Bloesem Remedies Nederland
Postbus 6139,
5960 AC Horst
The Netherlands
tel: 31 77 3987826
email: info@bloesem-remedies.com
website: www.bloesem-remedies.com

*Essences, courses, new practitioner and
training center. Website versions available
in English, Dutch, and German.*

This range is made mostly from the
plants and flowers growing in essence
practitioners Bram and Miep Zaalberg's
large organic garden at Horst, in the
Netherlands. Bram has been a
practitioner for 18 years, but now mostly
teaches about essences and healing. The
Zaalbergs began making essences —
including the first made from fungi — in
1986 and now have over 40, which are
sold internationally. They also run
seminars throughout the year.

Himalayan Flower Enhancers
PO Box 43, Central Tilba
NSW 2546, Australia
tel: 61 (0) 44 737 131
website: www.himalaya.com.au
Essences, videos, and teaching seminars.

These essences are made from the
unique flowers and plants growing in the
mighty Himalayas by developer Tanmaya,
who was raised on a farm by the sea in
southern Australia. He has also been a
landscape gardener, actor, counselor,
bodyguard, even a chef, as he wandered
the world in search of meaning,
immersing himself in different
psychotherapeutic, meditational, and
religious teachings, including the sacred
traditions of India.

Indigo Essences
The Yard Cottage
Dragonhold Stables
Timmore Lane
Newcastle, Co. Wicklow
Ireland
tel: 353 1 2011671
email: acall@indigo.ie
website: www.indigoessences.com

Essences and teaching seminars.

Indigo gem essence combinations for
children — also good for adults — were
developed by essence therapist and
homeopath Ann Callaghan, along with her
nephews Ben and Mica (age 10 and 11 at
the time) in County Wicklow, Ireland. Ann
originally trained as a homoeopath,

specializing in children, became Director of the Irish School of Homeopathy, and then began to make her essences in 1989. She now concentrates on these full-time, and teaches internationally.

Light Heart Essences
PO Box 35, Halesworth
Suffolk IP19 0WL, England
tel: 44 (0) 1986 785216
email: info@lightheartessences.co.uk
website: www.lightheartessences.co.uk

Essences, books, essence cards, consultations, and training courses.

This range of 56 essences is made in Suffolk, England, by therapist and healer Rose Titchiner from the energy of wildflowers, plants, and crystals. Besides being an essence developer and practitioner, Rose also runs workshops on emotional and spiritual healing, and flower essences. She is an author, the publisher of Waterlily Books, and a founder and executive committee member of the British Flower & Vibrational Essences Association.

Living Essences of Australia
PO Box 355, Scarborough
WA 6019, Australia

tel: 61 894 435 600
email: email@livingessences.com.au
website: www.livingessences.com.au

Essences, sprays, creams, and books, plus training (live and distance learning course to practitioner level) through the Living Flower Essences Academy of Australia (LiFE).

Perth-based Vasudeva and Kadambii Barnao, founders of the Australasian Flower Essence Academy, have developed their range over the last 25 years from the wildflowers of Western Australia. Over the last 20 years they have pioneered both essence research and the use of acupressure points and meridians as a method of applying essence therapy. This, and the development of their remedies into creams and lotions, has led to their work being taught and used in hospitals.

Living Tree Orchid Essences
Achamore House
Isle of Gigha
Argyll and Bute
Scotland PA41 7AD
tel: 44 (0) 1583 505385
email: flower@atlas.co.uk
website: www.healingflowers.com

Essences and color brochure. For courses, see IFER (page 300)

These essences are made from the energies of a collection of beautiful and delicate orchids originating from all over the world, but mostly from the tropics. No orchids are ever cut or harmed in any way to make the essences, which have been developed by Don Dennis of the International Flower Essence Repertoire and Heather Decam, with clairvoyant healer and lecturer Peter Tadd.

Pacific Essences
PO Box 8317, Victoria
British Columbia V8W 3R9
Canada
tel: 1 (250) 384 5560
email: info@pacificessences.com
website: www.pacificessences.com

Essences, sprays, and books, plus training courses worldwide.

Sabina Pettitt is an acupuncturist, counselor, essence therapist, and developer who is also trained in Ayurvedic medicine and Primordial Sound Meditation. She founded Pacific Essences in 1983. Her remedies are made from the energies of the plants and sea creatures of the wild NW Pacific Canadian coast. Sabina is based in Victoria BC, but travels the world teaching and speaking at conferences on natural therapy.

Petite Fleur Essences
Herbal Health Inc.
PO Box 330411, Forth Worth
Texas 76163, USA
tel: 1 (817) 293 5410
email: petitefl@aromahealthtexas.com
website: www.aromahealthtexas.com

Essences, books, video, natural skin care, aromatherapy blends, and healing floral waters, plus teaching seminars.

Dr. Judy Griffin is a fourth-generation flower-essence maker who has trained in Native American, Chinese, and Indian herbal traditions. A Master Herbalist with a PhD in Nutrition, she has written five books, and developed her essences in response to major health challenges faced by both herself and her children. Judy works with two cancer units in Texas and also teaches. Petite Fleur Essences are used by both orthodox and complementary practitioners worldwide.

South African Flower Essences
PO Box 721, Constantia
7847 Cape Town
South Africa
tel: 27 21 7946762
email: link via website
website: safloweressences.co.za

Essences and book.

These remedies are made from the wildflowers of South Africa's Table Mountain region — the place where leylines running the length of the continent converge, and which has always been held to be a powerful sacred site. The developer of the range is Jannet Unite-Penny, a lawyer by training who is also a mother and grandmother and has spent a lifetime working with metaphysics, natural medicine, and the interface between the two.

Wild Earth Animal Essences
PO Box 407, Charlottesville
VA 22902
USA
tel: 1 (434) 977 4615
email: info@animalessences.com
website: www.animalessences.com
Essences, animal cards, and teaching seminars.

These are made from the energies of wild animals through a process of meditation and ceremony in the wild, during which no animal is ever captured or harmed. The range's founder and developer, Daniel Mapel, is a Dartmouth graduate with a degree in Spiritual Psychology. He has worked as a wilderness guide in Wyoming and as a Peace Corps volunteer in Africa, and now practices in Virginia as a private counselor, working with survivors of childhood abuse.

Where to buy essences

If you would like to purchase an essence, or related items such as books or videos, from more than one maker, contact a mail-order distributor — this way, you will be able to get several essence ranges and many other products with a single phone call or email. Most sell to both the public and professionals.

Worldwide, there are many good, reliable mail-order companies, and major health retail outlets offering mail order.

A selection is listed below.

UNITED KINGDOM
The Cosmic Trader
76 Gillygate
York YO31 7EQ
tel: 44 (0) 1904 622706
email: essence@grayfin.net
website: www.cosmictrader.com
Good range of essences and books, and runs training courses in essence therapy with top international developers.

Fresh & Wild
stores countrywide
main office tel: 44 (0) 207 025 6030

Healthlines
tel: 44 (0) 1539 824099
email: admin@healthlines.co.uk
website: www.healthlines.co.uk
Excellent website and mail-order service, set up and run by a group of homeopaths and essence therapists. Wide range of essences from all over the world, plus herbal and homeopathic remedies, books, and flower cards. Runs courses and workshops in a Lake District setting. Offers an excellent money-saving service whereby they will make up an essence remedy of one or several different essences to order (so that you do not have to buy a number of single-essence bottles in order to make up a combination).

International Flower Essence Repertoire (IFER)
Achamore House
Isle of Gigha, Argyll and Bute
Scotland PA41 7AD
tel: 44 (0) 1583 505385
email: flower@atlas.co.uk
website: www.healingflowers.com
Wide range of many of the world's finest essences, books, and flower cards. Runs residential essence training courses with top international speakers, from their baronial manor house headquarters on a remote

Scottish island in the Inner Hebrides. Make
and distribute Living Tree Orchid Essences.

Napiers Dispensary

Glasgow
tel: 44 (0) 131 225 5542
(Bach Flower Remedies)

Neal's Yard Remedies

15 Neal's Yard
Covent Garden, London WC2H 9DP
(+ outlets all over London and countrywide)
tel: 44 (0) 207 379 7222
email: cservices@nealsyardremedies.com
website: www.nealsyardremedies.com
Sells flower essences, books, and a wide range
of natural health, beauty, herbal, and
aromatherapy products.

The Nutri Centre

7 Park Crescent, London W1B 1BF
tel: 44 (0) 207 436 5122
email: enq@nutricentre.com
website: www.nutricentre.com
Sells a comprehensive selection of international
flower essences and books, and a good range of
natural products such as herbs, supplements,
and homeopathic remedies. Shop in person at
their London store, or online.

Revital

tel: 44 (0) 800 252875
website: www.revital.com
(Bach Flower Remedies, and Australian
Bush Flower Essences)

Watkins Books

19 Cecil Court, Charing Cross Road
London WC2N 4EZ
tel: 44 (0) 20 7836 2182
email: service@watkinsbooks.com
website: www.watkinsbooks.com

AUSTRALIA

The International Flower Essence Centre (IFEC)

PO Box 1144, Hartwell VIC 3124, Melbourne
tel: 61 (0) 407 117 579
email: info@floweressences.com.au
website: www.floweressences.com.au
Offers a good mail-order service for several of
the world's finest essence ranges. Also produces
a newsletter.

You can also order essences direct from the
makers. If an essence maker is based
abroad, check their website, looking under
"Distributors." If there is one in your
country, it is worth ordering from them as
they will be able to supply you more quickly.

Further reading

General books on the subject:

Vibrational Medicine for the 21st Century
Richard Gerber, MD (Piatkus, 2000).

Anyone Can Dowse for Better Health Arthur
Bailey (Bailey, 1995).

The following are books about essences, by
the makers. Descriptions of the individual
essences and some catalogs are available on
their websites (see pages 293–99).

Alaskan Flower Essences *The Essence of
Healing: A Guide to Alaskan Essences* Steve
Johnson (The Alaskan Flower Essence
Project 1996, 2000).

Araretama Rainforest Essences *Araretama:
Rainforest Vibrational Healing Essences*
Sandra Epstein (Araretama).

Australian Bush Flower Essences *Australian
Bush Flower Essences* Ian White (Findhorn,
1993, 1998, Bantam 1991).
Bush Flower Healing Ian White (Bantam,
1999).

Bach Flower Remedies *Bach Flower Therapy:
The Complete Approach* Mechthild Scheffer
(Thorsons, 1990).

Bailey Flower Essences *The Bailey Flower
Essences Handbook* Arthur Bailey
(Bailey Flower Essences, 2000).

**Bloesem (Flower) Remedies of the
Netherlands** Extended booklet.

Findhorn Flower Essences *Findhorn Flower
Essences: Straight to the Heart of the Matter*
Marion Leigh (Findhorn Press, 1998).

Light Heart Essences *Truly Divine: Light
Heart Handbook & Inspirational Cards* Rose
Titchiner (Waterlily Books, 2004).

Living Essences of Australia *Australian
Flower Essences for the 21st Century* Vasudeva
and Kadambii Barnao (Australasian Flower
Essences Academy, 1997).

Pacific Essences *Energy Medicine: Healing
from the Kingdoms of Nature* Sabina Pettitt
(Pacific Essences, 1993, 1999).

South African Flower Essences *The South
African Flower Essences* Jannet Unite (South
African Flower & Gem Essences, 1995).

Petite Fleur Essences *The Healing Flowers*
Judy Griffin, PhD (Herbal Health Inc.,
2000).

Wild Earth Animal Essences *Into the Heart of
the Wild* Daniel Mapel, MA (Wild Earth,
2002).

Picture credits

2 Australian Bush Flower Essences; 3 Vasudeva and Kadambii Barnao/Living Flower Essence Academy of Australia; 7 Don Dennis/International Flower Essence Repertoire; 10 Richard Rockwood; 16 Australian Bush Flower Essences; 20 Arthur Bailey; 24-25 © Jacqui Hurst/GPL; 26-27 Steve Johnson/Alaskan Essences; 30-31 Andrew Lawson; 32-33 Australian Bush Flower Essences; 34-35 Pacific; 36-37 © GPL/James Guilliam; 40-41 Arthur Bailey; 42-43 Steve Johnson/Alaskan Essences; 44-45 Vasudeva and Kadambii Barnao/ Living Flower Essence Academy of Australia; 46-47 Australian Bush Flower Essences; 50 © JS Sira/GPL; 54-55 © Jerry Pavia/GPL; 56-57 Steve Johnson/Alaskan Essences; 58-59 © GPL/Howard Rice; 62-63 Don Dennis/International Flower Essence Repertoire; 64-65 D. Greig © Australian National Botanic Gardens; 66-67 Pacific Essences; 70 Jannet Unite-Penny/The South African Flower Essences; 74-75 Australian Bush Flower Essences; 76-77 GPL/Chris Burrows; 78-79 Steve Johnson/Alaskan Essences; 82-83 Arthur Bailey; 84-85 Pacific Essences; 86 © Rose Titchiner/Light Heart Essences; 90-91 Don Dennis/International Flower Essence Repertoire; 94-95 Australian Bush Flower Essences; 96-97 © M. Fagg, Australian National Botanic Gardens; 98-99 Steve Johnson/Alaskan Essences; 100 © JS Sira/GPL; 104-105 Australian Bush Flower Essences; 106-107 Pacific Essences; 108-109 Vasudeva and Kadambii Barnao/ Living Flower Essence Academy of Australia; 110-111 © Linda Burgess(Gardens & Plants)/GPL; 112-113 Steve Johnson/Alaskan Essences; 116 Araretama Bromeliad; 120-121 Australian Bush Flower Essences; 123-124 photolibrary.com/OSF; 125-126 Jocelen Janon - www.rosarosam.com; 128 © Rose Titchiner/Light Heart Essences; 132-133 © Juliette Wade/GPL; 134-135 D. Greig © Australian National Botanic Gardens; 141 © Andrew Lawson; 144 R. Hotchkiss © Australian National Botanic Gardens; 148-149 Australian Bush Flower Essences; 150 Steve Johnson/Alaskan Essences; 156-157 Arthur Bailey; 158-159 A. Lyne © Australian National Botanic Gardens; 160 © GPL/David Askham; 164-165 (above) © Juliette Wade/GPL (below) © GPL/Stephen Henderson; 166-167 © M. Fagg, Australian National Botanic Gardens; 168-169 Australian Bush Flower Essences; 172-173 Arthur Bailey; 174-175 © JS Sira/GPL; 176-177 © Rose Titchiner/Light Heart Essences; 178-179 Don Dennis/International Flower Essence Repertoire; 182 Australian Bush Flower Essences; 186-187 Andrea Jones/Garden ExposuresPhoto Library; 188-189 Vasudeva and Kadambii Barnao/ Living Flower Essence Academy of Australia; 190-191 © Mark Bolton/GPL; 192-193 photolibrary.com/OSF/Deni Bown; 194 Australian Bush Flower Essences; 198 Clay Perry; 200-201 Pacific Essences; 202-203 Arthur Bailey; 204-205 Findhorn Flower Essences; 208-211 Don Dennis/International Flower Essence Repertoire; 212-213 Steve Johnson/Alaskan Essences; 218-219 Australian Bush Flower Essences; 220-221 © Andrew Lawson; 224 Jocelen Janon - www.rosarosam.com; 228-229 Arthur Bailey; 230-231 (left) © Andrew Lawson; 230-231 (right)Marianne Majerus; 232-233 Australian Bush Flower Essences; 236 © GPL/David Cavagnaro; 240-241 photolibrary.com/OSF/Tim Shepherd; 242-243 © Rex Butcher/GPL; 244-245 Australian Bush Flower Essences; 246-247 Pacific Essences; 250 © Ron Sutherland/GPL; 252-253 © Sunniva Harte/GPL; 254-255 Pacific Essences; 258-259 Steve Johnson/Alaskan Essences; 260-1 Arthur Bailey; 262 © GPL/Bjorn Forsberg; 266-267 Australian Bush Flower Essences; 270-271 © Melanie Eclare; 272-273 © JS Sira/GPL; 276 Australian Bush Flower Essences; 280 Arthur Bailey.

Author acknowledgments

Very many grateful thanks to the 17 essence producers from all over the world who helped with this book — we could not have produced it without all your marvelous feedback, cooperation, and fantastic photographs.

I'd also like to thank Mac McKean for all his help, Anne Furniss for her vision and enthusiasm, Ros Holder for her great design and, with the help of Sam Rolfe, her tireless picture research; and the earth's glorious wealth of plants, flowers, natural environments, and their devas for allowing their energy to be used in essence form.

Especial thanks to our two terrific Editorial Consultants, Beth Tyers and Rose Titchiner, for your invaluable advice and suggestions:

Beth Tyers is an experienced homeopath, flower essence practitioner, and healer. A senior lecturer and manager at Lakeland College of Homeopathy in England's beautiful Lake District, she has practices both there and in central London, besides running healing retreats and group seminars at her home in the Lakes. Beth teaches all over the UK as well as internationally (Iceland, Egypt, Ireland) and is currently completing a book developing education about flower essences.

Rose Titchiner is an essence developer, flower essence therapist, and healer-practitioner based in Suffolk, England. Her range, Light Heart, is made from the energy of wild flowers, plants, and crystals. Rose runs workshops on emotional/ spiritual healing and essences, is an author, and is the publisher of Waterlily Books. She is also a founder member and executive committee member of the British Flower & Vibrational Essences Association, and a member of the British Association of Flower Essence Producers.